Surface Anatomy for
Radiographers

Surface Anatomy for Radiographers

D. W. McKears, BA, DCR
Principal of the Gwent School of Radiography

and

R. H. Owen, MD, DMR
Consultant Radiologist, Royal Gwent Hospital;
Director of the Gwent School of Radiography

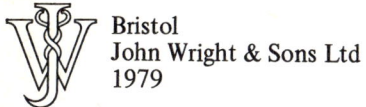
Bristol
John Wright & Sons Ltd
1979

CIP Data
McKears, D W
    Surface anatomy for radiographers.
    1. Anatomy, Human   2. Radiography, Medical
    I. Title   II. Owen, R H
    611   QM23.2

ISBN 0 7236 0511 4

Reprinted 1980

PRINTED IN GREAT BRITAIN BY
JOHN WRIGHT & SONS LTD, AT THE STONEBRIDGE PRESS,
BRISTOL

Preface

A sound knowledge of surface markings has always been necessary for accurate radiography, as most of the radiographic centring points have been based on surface anatomy.

The advent of ultrasound has increased this need, and even experienced radiographers have found it necessary to improve their knowledge of the position of the abdominal organs, before undertaking ultrasound examinations.

We hope that the present volume will be of value not only to students of radiography, but also to ultrasound technicians and radiologists by providing a convenient handbook for easy reference.

The book has been arranged in two parts, the first dealing with bony landmarks and surface features of particular value in radiographic positioning or in any of the newer scanning techniques.

The second part is concerned with the surface markings of the internal organs, structures and vessels, with specialized examination techniques particularly in mind.

Newport, Gwent   D. W. McK.
1979   R. H. O.

Acknowledgements

We are indebted to Professor D. B. Moffat, of the Anatomy Department, University College, Cardiff, for help with anatomical terminology and anatomical details, also to Mrs O. Palmer, of the Royal Gwent Hospital Postgraduate Department, for her patient and invaluable help in typing the manuscript.

We thank the following for permission to reproduce prints from their publications and collections:
The Victoria and Albert Museum (Crown Copyright).
Fratelli Alinari, Florence.
The Mansell Collection.
Faber & Faber Ltd and Professor R. D. Lockhart.

Our particular thanks must go to Mr A. J. Bezear of the Audio-Visual Services Department of Nottingham University Medical School for his patience and skill in producing the really excellent drawings for the line illustrations.

We would like to thank Mr Kingham and Dr Emerson of John Wright & Sons Ltd, for their help during the preparation and publication of this book.

Contents

List of Plates (between pp. 40 and 41)

Plate 1. Posterior view of neck and shoulder.

Plate 2. Anterior view of chin and neck, chin raised and muscles set. *(Reproduced by permission of Faber & Faber Ltd from 'Living Anatomy' by Professor R. D. Lockhart.)*

Plate 3. Anterior view of thorax. *(Reproduced by permission of the Mansell Collection, London: Print from Fratelli Alinari, Florence (Michaelangelo's David).)*

Plate 4. Anterior view of abdomen. *(Reproduced by permission of the Mansell Collection, London: Print from Fratelli Alinari, Florence (Michaelangelo's David).)*

Plate 5. Shoulder region, posterior view. *(Reproduced by permission of the Victoria and Albert Museum.)*

Plate 6. Forearm and hand. *(Reproduced by permission of the Victoria and Albert Museum.)*

Plate 7. Lumbar spine and trunk. *(Reproduced by permission of the Victoria and Albert Museum.)*

Plate 8. Thigh, anterior view. *(Reproduced by permission of the Victoria and Albert Museum.)*

Plate 9. Lower leg and calf. *(Reproduced by permission of the Victoria and Albert Museum.)*

Plate 10. Axilla. Triceps extending elbow against resistance. Note biceps running into axilla posterior to pectoralis major, and the position of the neurovascular bundle. *(Reproduced by permission of Faber & Faber Ltd from 'Living Anatomy' by Professor R. D. Lockhart.)*

Part 1

Surface anatomy of bony structures

Chapter 1

Reference points and terminology

In order to describe the positions of structures and organs within the body we need a framework of reference points and a generally-accepted terminology. For descriptive purposes it is usual to accept the traditional convention of a body in an erect position, feet together and facing forwards, arms by the sides with palms forward. This is known as the *anatomical position.*

ASPECTS OF THE BODY
TERMINOLOGY

The front of the body is termed its *anterior* aspect, the back view its *posterior* aspect and the view from either side the *right* or *left lateral* aspect. An upper aspect of a part of the body is termed *superior*, a view from below, *inferior*. Neither of these terms carries any implication of quality and the terms have only positional significance. The aspects of the hand tend to be termed *palmar* instead of anterior, and *dorsal* instead of posterior. The aspects of the foot are termed *dorsal* and *plantar* instead of superior and inferior. The term *proximal* is applied to parts nearer the heart, *distal* being taken to mean further from the heart. A part of the lower leg below the knee would be considered proximal whereas one nearer the ankle would be considered distal.

PLANES AND LINES

Imagine a plane passing longitudinally through the body dividing it into right and left halves. This is termed the *median plane*. A line drawn down the front of the body where the

1

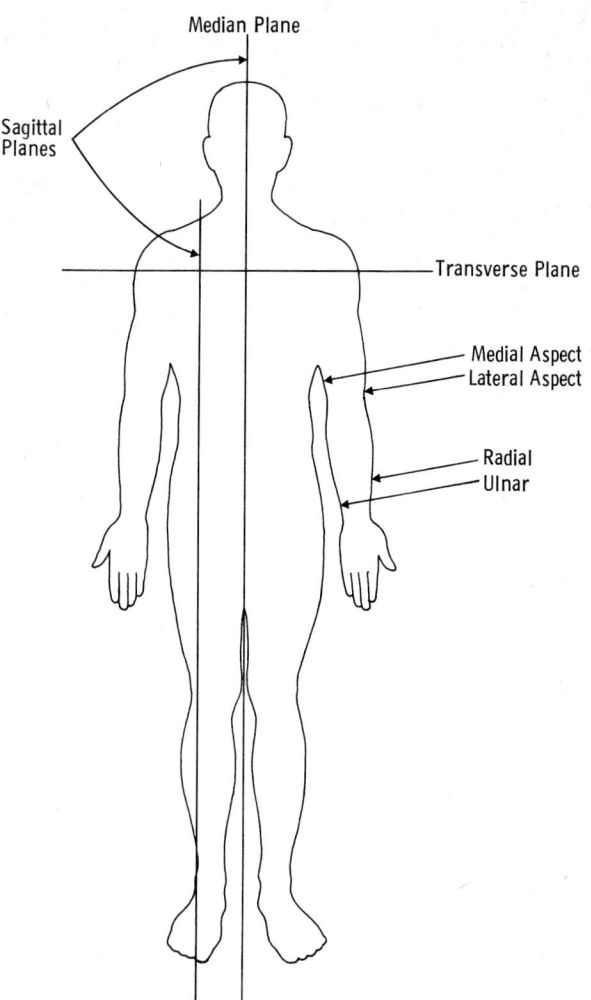

Fig. 1. Body planes; anterior view.

median plane cuts it is called the *anterior median line* and a similar line drawn where the median plane cuts the posterior surface of the body is called the *posterior median line*. Any plane parallel to the median plane is termed a *sagittal plane* and will run parallel to the sagittal suture of the skull from which it takes its name (*Fig.* 1).

Any vertical plane at right angles to the median plane is called a *coronal plane* after the coronal suture of the skull to which it runs approximately parallel. Any plane at right angles to both median and coronal planes simultaneously is a *horizontal* plane which will divide the body into superior and inferior portions (*Fig.* 2).

POSTURE

We must remember that whilst we use the conventional anatomical position already mentioned and described for nomenclature purposes, it is not a practical position for clinical examination. The body may be placed in a variety of postures, *supine* meaning lying on the back, *prone* face downwards, *decubitus* meaning lying on one side. These are the commonest met postural terms other than *erect*, which is self explanatory. The reason for the need to mention the posture of the body is mainly due to gravitational effect on some organs so that their positions relative to bony structures may vary.

THE AVERAGE SUBJECT

Although the relative positions of some parts of the body vary little from one subject to another this is not always so, especially in the case of some thoracic and many abdominal organs. Descriptions usually assume an *average* subject, but allowances will have to be made for differences arising from *subject type, sex, age, state of health, muscular tone* and *physical development*, the effects of which can with a little experience be intelligently and accurately anticipated.

LANDMARKS

The landmarks of the body vary greatly in usefulness.

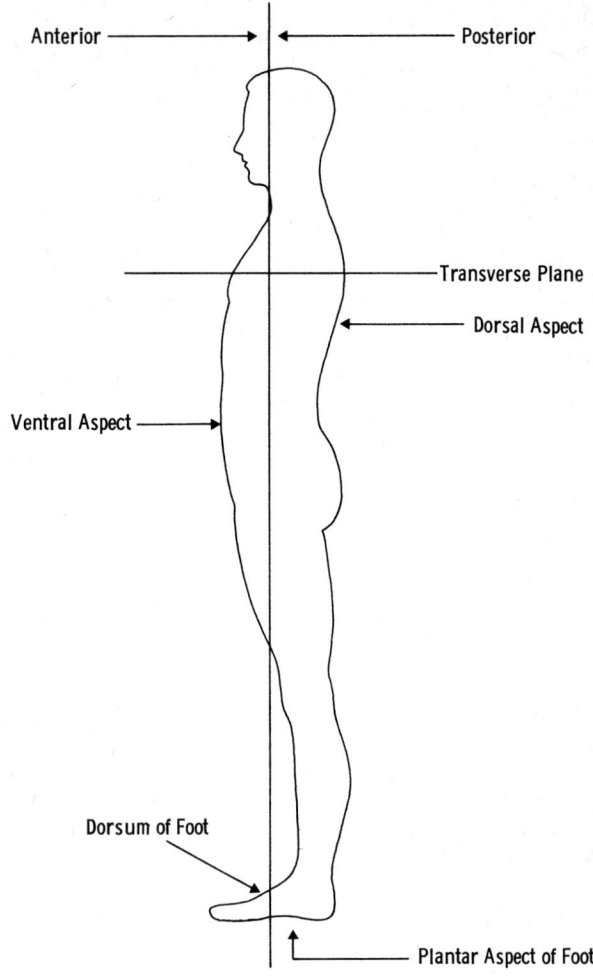

Fig. 2. Body planes; lateral view.

Essentially they are consistently found prominent body features with a known reliably constant relationship to adjacent deeper structures. They may be used as a guide to the position of deeper structures, the location of which is difficult to ascertain by other clinical methods.

BONY LANDMARKS

These are particularly useful because of their constant and predictable relationship to each other and because they form a convenient network of landmarks covering most parts of the body. The position of most structures can usually be described in relation to them.

SOFT-TISSUE LANDMARKS

These are in general less useful than bony ones because of their variability in relationship not only to each other but to other bony prominences. However, a soft-tissue landmark such as the *umbilicus* may be almost useless in localizing a specific vertebral level for radiographic purposes but serves well as an idiosyncratic reference point in echography.

The *outer canthus* of the *eye*, although undeniably a soft-tissue landmark is quite constant in its relationship with the bony orbit and may be used with confidence whereas the female nipple is of very limited localizing value.

Scars, lines and *acquired markings* may occasionally prove useful. The presence of *surgical scars* may indicate disarrangement of or absence of an organ. The use of *temporary lines* marked on a patient's skin may facilitate repeated accurate placing of treatment applicators in radiotherapy. The use of pre-existing *tattoo* markings may be of limited value once their relationships are accurately established in that individual.

PALPATION AND INSPECTION

As a preliminary to grasping surface relationships it is essential that one becomes familiar with the main body landmarks and learns how to *palpate* (which means to locate by manual pressure) and how to facilitate *visual inspection* to avoid distress to the subject. *Palpation* must never be more forceful than is necessary, but must be conducted with warm hands using the fingertips for revealing smaller structures only and the palm of the hand or its medial border for more prominent ones. It must be remembered that some structures can only be clearly identified when overlying muscle is relaxed and this necessitates care in choice of subject posture during palpation. Muscular structures themselves will usually be more readily identified when suitably tensed. *Visual inspection* may call for the use of simple aids if it is to be fully effective. These may include a small electric torch with a lens-ended lamp, disposable tongue depressors and a small dental mirror for intra-oral work. Visual inspection is invariably aided by good general lighting conditions and a clear field of view. Before considering the merits of any surface marking or bony landmark of the trunk it is appropriate to mention the influence of general body type – whether average, small, thickset or elongated – on the relative positions of bony and other structures. This effect may be quite considerable, causing the same part to appear at a variety of vertebral levels in differing subjects. This does not necessarily diminish the value of a landmark but it does indicate that whilst it may be used with confidence for some purposes, it may need to be treated with caution for others. The factors causing the variation are evident to the careful observer as are also the effects of varying *muscle tone* which may have similar influence. Before proceeding to a systematic exploration of the major bony landmarks the following small exercise may help to give the student an understanding of what can be achieved by the use of the simple methods outlined. As when locating any bony landmarks, the part should first be identified on a skeleton using any of the well-illustrated anatomical reference books (Gray, Cunningham etc.) and then on the student's own body.

It is suggested that for this exercise we use an area with which we have considerable familiarity and in which we are all expert in detecting quite small variations. The face, which we use for recognition purposes in others at once makes us aware

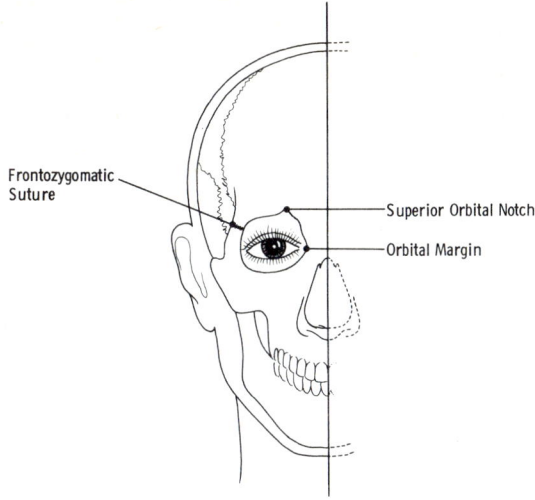

Fig. 3. Orbital margins.

that although there are great general similarities between individuals there are also great ranges of readily noted minor variations. We must expect this level of variation to produce close approximations rather than perfect accuracy in our work, but at the same time we can build up confidence in knowing what we can reasonably expect to achieve.

PRELIMINARY EXERCISE

The *inferior orbital margin*, readily recognized on the dried skull, is easily accessible to palpation in the living subject. Following it laterally and upwards, the fingertip, or even an area as large as the end of the thumb will quite easily locate the position of the *frontozygomatic* suture, an apparently very small detail which being superficially placed is quite prominent. If the finger now follows the underside of the *superior orbital margin* pressing upwards it will be found possible, but rather less easy, to locate the *superior orbital notch* at a position about 3 cm ($1\frac{3}{16}$ in) from the midline (*Fig.* 3).

This small exercise, carefully followed, indicates that provided we know for what we are looking even quite small details can be identified if they are superficially placed. But what of deeper structures not accessible to direct palpation? If they are known to have a consistent relationship to other prominent but otherwise unremarkable structures, then their position can be deduced. We shall, therefore need to take note of some structures which are of only scant intrinsic interest but usefully prominent, as well as others whose significance is more immediate.

With this in mind we shall now turn to a general survey of some of the more readily available bony surface markings used as landmarks.

Chapter 2

The skull

SKULL LINES AND PLANES

Unless radiography of the skull is undertaken in a carefully standardized manner the films produced are needlessly difficult to compare with others, and small but significant differences may be missed. Head and facial shapes display notable idiosyncratic differences and variations which might seem to make standardized positioning impractical. There are fortunately sufficient common features between all skulls to permit systematic positioning and comparison by use of various lines and planes based on consistently related prominent features. The radiographer clearly needs an intelligent appreciation of how this can be applied in practice.

The anatomist, able to compare dried skulls at leisure, tends to use the *anthropological baseline* (infra-orbital meatal line), a line drawn from the *lower orbital margin* to the upper part of the external *auditory meatus*. This is also known as the *Frankfort* line and also *Reid's baseline*. In the living subject the use of this baseline presents problems since one has to palpate to locate the lower orbital margin rather than to see it easily and this reduces its value in difficult clinical situations (*Fig.* 4).

The radiographer tends to find another line, the *orbito-meatal baseline*, more convenient because it is easily visualized in almost any clinical situation.

Fortunately it has a quite predictable variation of around 10° from the anthropological baseline so that when a positioning method referring vaguely to 'the baseline' is tried experimentally and proves disappointing it may be assumed

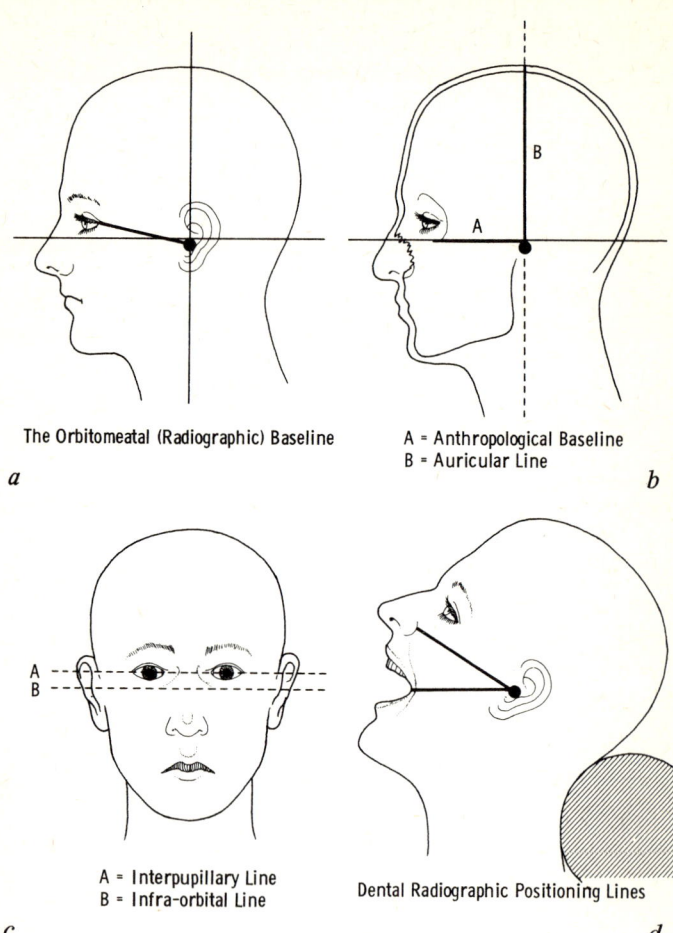

The Orbitomeatal (Radiographic) Baseline

A = Anthropological Baseline
B = Auricular Line

a

b

A = Interpupillary Line
B = Infra-orbital Line

Dental Radiographic Positioning Lines

c

d

Fig. 4. Base lines of skull. *a*, Radiographic baseline. *b*, Anthropological baseline (infra-orbital meatal line). *c*, Interpupillary line. *d*, Dental positioning lines.

that the alternative baseline was intended and correction applied.

A further reason for the radiographer's interest in the orbitomeatal baseline lies in another line which may be drawn about 2·5 cm (1 in) above and parallel to it. This imaginary line will be found to join the glabella to the external auditory meatus and cuts across the position of the roof of the orbit, the anterior clinoid processes, and the highest part of the petrous bones.

The position of the following non-palpable structures can be judged with sufficient accuracy to enable good coned projections to be made as follows:

PITUITARY FOSSA

A point measured about 2·5 cm (1 in) in front of and 2·5 cm (1 in) above the external auditory meatus will indicate the position of the fossa from the lateral aspect and is commonly used as a radiographic centring point for it in lateral projections (*Fig.* 4).

PINEAL GLAND

A point about 3 cm ($1\frac{3}{16}$ in) above and 1·5 cm ($\frac{5}{8}$ in) behind the external auditory meatus indicates the normal position from the lateral aspect.

FORAMEN MAGNUM

A point about 2·0 cm ($\frac{3}{4}$ in) below and 0·5–1·0 cm ($\frac{3}{16}-\frac{3}{8}$ in) behind the external auditory meatus when the orbitomeatal baseline is horizontal indicates the position of the anterior border of the foramen from the lateral aspect.

The use of the *interpupillary line* is invaluable in arranging lateral projections (*Fig.* 4).

The ready availability of such lines on which a positioning aid such as a protractor can be aligned makes repeated accurate positioning easier. Using the bony landmarks from which distances to centring points can be measured further assists in obtaining standardized projections.

In dental radiography the features which might seem the obvious ones to use as landmarks may be either absent or obscured due to clinical conditions and two imaginary lines, generally known as the *upper* and *lower dental positioning lines,* are found most useful. These involve use of soft-tissue structures but are found to be both consistently reliable and easily seen in almost any clinical situation (*Fig.* 4).

The upper line, which is parallel to, but *not* coincident with the *upper occlusal plane* (i.e. a plane drawn through the biting surfaces of the upper teeth when present) is drawn from the *ala* of the *nose* to the *tragus* of the *ear*. The lower line is drawn from the *corner* of the *mouth* to the *tragus* of the *ear* and as might by now be expected is parallel to, but *not* coincident with, the *lower occlusal plane.* Consultation with any sound book on dental radiography will show that the use of these lines is quite basic to successful dental radiographic technique since X-ray beam angulation to obtain undistorted projections is based on horizontal (or in some circumstances, vertical) alignment of each line in turn according to whether upper or lower jaw is being worked upon.

SURFACE FEATURES OF THE HEAD ACCESSIBLE TO VISUAL INSPECTION AND PALPATION

It is suggested that the earlier exercise exploring the bony region of the eye is now repeated and extended to cover the whole of the head and neck region (*Figs.* 5 and 6).

Starting at the lower orbital margin a finger gently palpates working laterally along the curve and then ascending. At a point about 1 cm (⅜ in) lateral to and slightly above the *lateral canthus* of the *eye* (the outer junction of upper and lower lids) a small circular movement of the finger will detect an irregularity in bony outline at the *frontozygomatic suture.* A change in bony character will be noted as the finger follows what has become the *superior orbital margin*. The sharp ridge which characterizes the inferior and lateral orbital margins is replaced by a less regular edge, broken in outline at the *superior orbital notch* which can usually be felt at about the

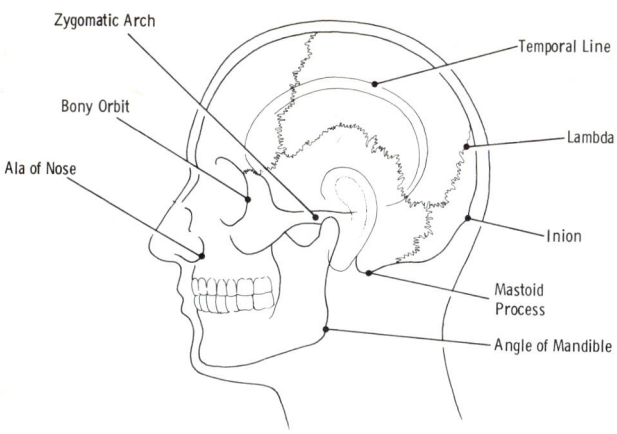

Fig. 5. Lateral skull.

highest point of the curve of the *superior orbital margin* (*Fig.* 3). Occasionally, due to a variation in which the notch becomes bridged it becomes very difficult to locate. A finger rolled above the eyebrow will detect the *superciliary ridge* of that side forming with the other, part of the *superciliary arch.* It will be noted that this is a feature which varies considerably in prominence from one subject to another. The *glabella* will be recognized as a flattened midline area between the two superciliary ridges. It is one of two landmarks between which the radiographic centring point for the lateral projection of skull is located. About 2·5 cm (1 in) below it in a well marked depression above the nose is the *nasion*, the junction of the frontal and nasal bones. Because it lies in a depression it can be used as a stabilizing and fixing reference point in a device called a *craniostat* used for precise and readily repeatable positioning of the skull during its radiographic examination for recording growth changes. The nasion is also used as a radiographic centring point (*Fig.* 6).

The *nasal bones* can be readily traced out between the

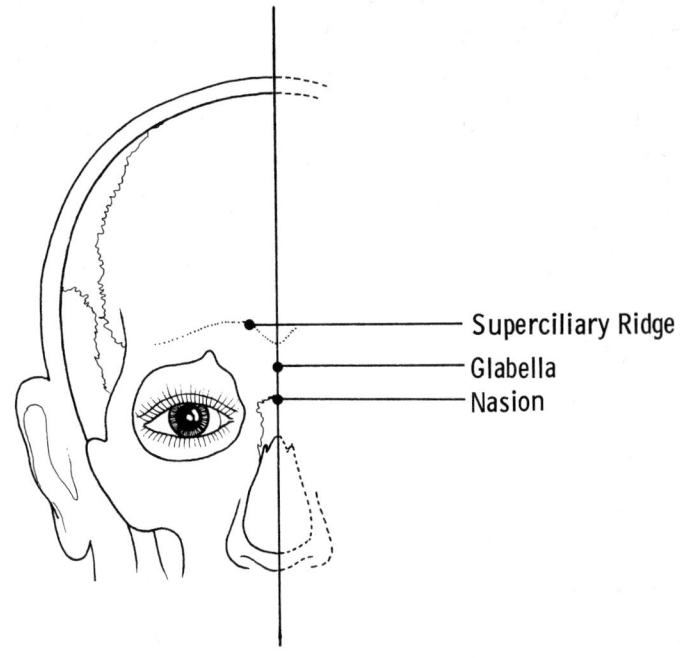

Fig. 6. Frontal region of face.

finger and thumb to their irregular termination a little way down the nose. The cartilaginous prolongation of the bony *nasal septum* can be moved from side to side to a limited extent below this level. The position of the superior opening of the *nasolacrimal canal* will be suggested rather than distinctly felt by a finger pressing gently slightly behind the *medial canthus* of the closed eye (*Fig.* 7). If the finger now continues downwards and laterally along the *maxillary margin* of the *orbit*, a small irregularity in outline will be noted corresponding to the position of the suture between *maxilla* and *zygoma*. The *infra-orbital foramen*, transmitting the *infra-orbital nerve* and vessels lies at a point about 0·5 cm ($\frac{3}{16}$ in)

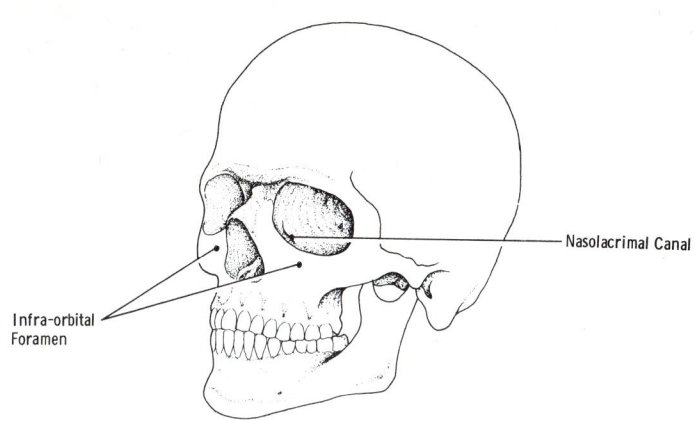

Nasolacrimal Canal

Infra-orbital
Foramen

Fig. 7. Skull: orbits and lacrimal canal.

below this but somewhat nearer the nose (*Fig.* 7) It may
be felt only indistinctly in most subjects. If the finger then
continues laterally to the midpoint of the curve of the
zygomatic portion of the *orbital margin* and is then moved
about 2·0 cm (¾ in) below the margin it should be possible to
make out the position of the *zygomaticofacial foramen.*

Exploration of the area above the upper lip will reveal
palpable vertical ridging of the maxilla due to tooth sockets
where dentition persists. Of these ridges the most notable
corresponds to the position of the root of the upper canine
tooth and is termed the *canine eminence*. Above it there is a
wide shallow depression extending close to the level of the
orbital margin and termed the *canine fossa*. A finger placed
horizontally and pressed upwards and posteriorly against the
nose from below will detect the *anterior nasal spine,* a midline
structure arising at the junction of the maxillae.

SURFACE FEATURES OF THE LATERAL ASPECT OF THE HEAD

The general position of the *zygomatic arch* can be made out easily on palpation and it is not particularly difficult to palpate its lower border using firm pressure although palpation is a little impeded by the attachment of the masseter muscle. The *upper border* of the *zygomatic arch*, an obvious feature on a dried skull, is disappointingly difficult to palpate. It can be felt anteriorly at its angular function with the *posterior margin* of the *frontal process* of the *zygoma* (*Fig. 5*). If the fingers now work upwards and then laterally and posteriorly the *temporal line* may be traced out passing across the skull and then coming downwards and finally forwards again to join the *supramastoid crest* behind the ear. If the flat of the hand is used to palpate an area above and behind the highest posterior portion of the temporal line the *parietal eminence* will be found easily. The position of the *pre-auricular point* on the posterior root of the zygomatic arch immediately in front of the point of attachment of the auricle can be verified on light pressure by picking up pulsation of the *superficial temporal artery* overlying the bone (*see* p. 52). The rest of the *posterior root* of the *zygomatic arch* lies beneath the auricle through which it can be felt on deep pressure. A finger placed in front of the tragus of the ear pushing upwards and a little backwards will find the *head* of the *mandible* when the jaw is made to perform side to side movements. The *mastoid process* can be palpated more easily when the auricle is pulled forward and the finger directed upwards immediately below and behind the attachment of the ear (*Fig. 5*).

The external auditory meati are most useful landmarks for the radiographer, as points from which to arrange positioning guidelines, as reference points from which to locate centring points (temporomandibular joints, sella turcica, mastoid process etc.) and as a means of precise fixing of a head within one of the various types of craniostat for radiographic use.

REGION OF THE BACK OF THE SKULL

The most obvious feature of the back of the skull is the *external occipital protuberance*, the centre of which is termed the *inion*. It is of great value to the radiographer because of the absence of other features of consistent prominence in that area. Despite this it can be missed or seem hard to find by the inexperienced unless palpated by an upward stroke along the neck towards the back of the head when it can be felt unmistakably. Since it is a point from which it is usual to measure various radiographic centring points and may also be used as a location point when using some types of craniostat the radiographer must be able to find it unhesitatingly.

Except on dried skulls from very elderly subjects it is usually easy to see the *lambda*, the point at which the lambdoid and sagittal sutures meet. It can be identified easily in the living by using the flat of the hand to locate the slight depression in which it lies some 7·5 cm (3 in) above the inion, along the skull surface (*Fig.* 5). The position of the *sagittal suture* can be recognized readily in many subjects as a central slight furrow along the top of the head meeting the *coronal suture* at a point called the *bregma*. This can be found just in front of the imaginary *auricular line* as it reaches the top of the skull (*Fig.* 5). In infants the bregma is represented by a four-sided area about 3·75 cm ($1\frac{1}{2}$ in) anteroposteriorly 2·5 cm (1 in) across. This is called the *anterior fontanelle* and it can be seen to pulsate in time with the heartbeat in small babies. Closure is complete by the middle of the second year of life (18 months normally). The lambda is represented in infants by a three-sided area called the *posterior fontanelle* which closes normally by the end of the second month of life. Both anterior and posterior fontanelles are areas of fibrous membrane which have yet to ossify and which are commonly referred to as 'soft spots' and form almost visible features when not hair-covered.

Chapter 3

The mouth and lower jaw

When the mouth and lips remain closed and the face is relaxed, the junction of the upper and lower lips is fairly constantly related to the interval between the 1st and 2nd premolar teeth despite considerable variation in lip size and shape. That part of the mouth which may be explored by a finger inserted between the lips when the teeth are clenched firmly is called the *vestibule* of the *mouth*. Within it the surface of the *maxilla* superiorly, and inferiorly, the *anterior border* of the mandible including the *coronoid process* of the *ramus* of the *mandible* can be palpated. It will be noted that the mandibular surface is notably ridged over the root of each incisor tooth, and particularly so over the roots of the canine teeth. In areas where teeth have been lost or extracted the *alveolar margin*, the tooth-supporting area of the jaw, will be reduced in prominence in proportion to the length of time the teeth have been absent.

On opening the mouth to a comfortable rather than a widely opened degree, the teeth, when present, can be more fully examined.

At birth, no teeth are in evidence but the first set of teeth, later to be shed, appears at very approximately the times given in the table opposite, though considerable variations may occasionally be noted. In general girls are in advance of boys in dates of erupting teeth. There are 20 teeth in the deciduous dentition, 10 in each jaw.

TERMINOLOGY AND THE DENTAL X-RAY REQUEST FORMULA
Teeth nearer the front of the mouth are termed *proximal* whereas those further back are termed *distal*. The surface of a tooth facing the vestibule of the mouth is termed *buccal*;

ERUPTION OF DECIDUOUS TEETH

	Age in months
Lower central incisors	6−9
Upper incisors	8−10
Lower lateral incisors	15−21
First molars	15−21
Canines	16−20
Second molars	20−24

The permanent dentition replaces the deciduous dentition after eruption of the first permanent molars. The sequence and approximate timing is:

	Age in years
First molars	Around 6
Central incisors	After 7
Lateral incisors	After 8
First premolars	After 9
Second premolars	After 10
Canines	After 11
Second molars	After 12
Third molars	After 17
	but may appear very late even after 25

that facing the tongue, *lingual*. The neighbouring edges of the proximal teeth are termed *medial* or *lateral* according to location. In the case of the distal teeth which tend to be more obviously four-sided the terms *anterior* (or *proximal*) and *posterior* (or *distal*) are used to describe forward or rearward-facing surfaces respectively. For dental X-ray request form purposes, the deciduous dentition is referred to by a formula of alphabetically consecutive letters, a to e, indicating tooth positions as seen from the *buccal* (outward facing) aspect. The full formula, only half of which is shown in *Fig.* 8 is:

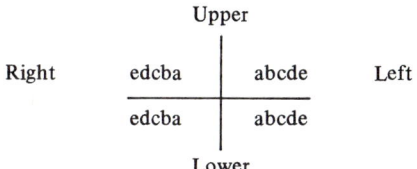

```
                     Upper
                       |
   Right      edcba    |    abcde      Left
                       |
             edcba     |    abcde
                       |
                     Lower
```

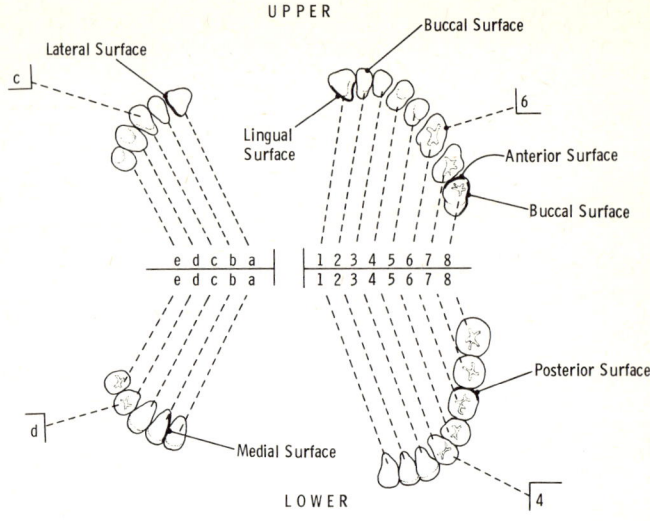

Fig. 8. Dental formula.

In practice the explanatory words shown above are omitted and when less than a complete survey or even less than a whole quadrant of a jaw is to be examined a further abbreviation may be used e.g.

From *Fig.* 8 c⌋ one sees that a view of the right upper canine is required in a child. d̄⌋ refers to the child's right lower first molar.

Figures from 1 to 8 are used to indicate teeth in the permanent dentition.

The key to each system is:

DECIDUOUS   a Central incisor
                    b Lateral incisor
                    c Canine
                    d First molar
                    e Second molar

PERMANENT   1   Central incisor
                   2   Lateral incisor
                   3   Canine
                   4   First premolar
                   5   Second premolar
                   6   First molar
                   7   Second molar
                   8   Third molar

From *Fig.* 8 it will be seen that $\underline{6}$ represents a request for a
view of the first left upper molar and $\overline{4}$ a first left lower
premolar.

The *hard palate*, formed by the *palatine process* of the
maxilla and posteriorly the *palatine bones*, can be felt on
upward pressure to the roof of the mouth but the individual
bones cannot be seperately identified. Medially and posteriorly
to the posterior termination of the alveolar region (upper) it is
possible to feel the *hamular process* of the *sphenoid*. A finger
following the medial aspect of the mandible posteriorly and
upwards will detect its *coronoid process*. The position of the
temporomandibular joint can be located readily by placing a
finger just in front of the tragus of the ear and making side-to-
side movements of the jaw. The forward sliding movement of
the joint on opening the mouth can then be examined more
easily once the position of the joint has been established. The
posterior margin of the *ramus* of the *mandible* is more readily
palpable in its lower part below the level of the lobe of the ear.
The very prominent *angle* of the *mandible* should be noted.
Though slightly less prominent in the female it is always easily
found and is a useful guide to the level of the body of the
third cervical vertebra. The inferior margin of the mandible is
easy to palpate over its whole length. It is possible to feel a
ridge in the anterior midline position of the jaw marking the
position of the *symphysis menti.* Below the *mental protuberance* a slight notch can be felt marking on the anterior
aspect of the lower margin of the jaw the union of its two
halves. About 2·5 cm (1 in) to either side of this the *mental*

tubercles are found if two fingers are suitably placed close together and moved about pushing a little upwards from below the margin of the jaw (*Figs.* 5 and 9).

Chapter 4

The neck

POSTERIOR ASPECT

A finger exploring the midline region about two finger spaces below the inion will encounter the *spinous processes* of the *cervical vertebrae*, that of the second being the first prominence recognized. There can be considerable difficulty in identifying with certainty the spinous processes of the middle cervical region, even when the head is bent forward to increase separation between them. The obvious prominence in the midline nearer shoulder level is the spinous process of the 7th cervical vertebra with an almost equal (occasionally even more obvious) prominence just below it representing the spinous process of the first thoracic vertebra. In the child the spinous processes of the cervical region lie in a clearly-defined median furrow which becomes obscured towards adulthood (*Plate* 1).

ANTERIOR ASPECT

The most prominent bony feature of the upper anterior part of the neck is the *hyoid bone* which can be gently gripped between finger and thumb as it lies just below the mandible. It can be felt to rise during swallowing movements. Below it and more prominent in males is the *prominence* of the *thyroid cartilage*, commonly known as the 'Adam's Apple'. Its position can be seen when the head is allowed to fall back. Careful palpation will permit recognition of most parts of the cartilage but practice is best gained on a male subject. Below this it is possible to make out the *cricoid cartilage* (*Fig.* 9) and the *trachea* to the point where it becomes inaccessible below the deep depression between the sternal end of the clavicles at the *suprasternal notch*. The thumb pressing downwards in the sternal notch rests on the upper border of the *manubrium*

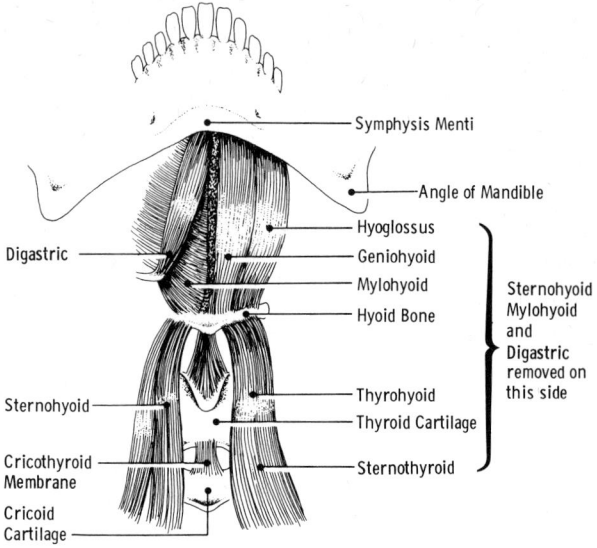

Fig. 9. Cartilages of neck.

sterni. It should be noted that some of the anterior structures of the neck can be made to reveal their positions visually against the stretched skin of the extended neck (*Plate* 2).

LATERAL ASPECT

Deep pressure at a point about 1·0 cm (⅜ in) below and in front of the tip of the mastoid process will detect the *transverse process* of the *atlas vertebra*. A point 2·5 cm (1 in) behind the angle of the jaw when the subject maintains the neck in a normally relaxed position is a reliable guide to the position of the body of the 3rd cervical vertebra and is important as the accepted radiographic centring point for the lateral projection of the cervical region.

Chapter 5

The thorax

ANTERIOR ASPECT

The upper border of the *manubrium sterni* is not as constant in vertebral level as some elementary textbooks seem to imply, even in quiet respiration. Its range of movement between full inspiration and full expiration varies between individuals; its position in stockily-built subjects tends to be higher in quiet respiration. Raising the arms above shoulder level accompanied by a stretching movement upwards will raise sternal level considerably. Type of breathing, whether costal or abdominal will also contribute to variation in sternal level. The range of inspiratory variation can be as much as 2—4 cm ($\frac{3}{4}$—$1\frac{1}{2}$ in) above the quiet-breathing position, full expiratory variation being about 2·0 cm ($\frac{3}{4}$ in) below. This may be slightly further affected by body position, whether erect or supine, and by age, notably in the elderly subject whose chest has taken on the characteristic barrel-type conformation raising the anterior thoracic levels relative to spine.

In an average subject in quiet respiration the floor of the sternal notch lies at the level of intervertebral disc T2—T3. The *sternoclavicular joint* is an almost visible structure in thin subjects and readily palpable. The whole anterior and superior surface of the clavicle can be palpated (*Plate* 3). Because its length is easily determined, vertical arbitrary lines from its midpoint or the junctions of its thirds are easily drawn to facilitate topographical description of the anterior part of the thorax. Careful palpation of the clavicle near the shoulder will reveal the position of the anteriorly-facing *acromioclavicular joint* which is often rather illogically expected to be found at the point of the shoulder.

There can be occasional difficulty in finding the position of the *sternal angle,* the junction of the body and the manubrium. The sternal angle is referred to in some books as the *Angle of Ludwig* and also as the *Angle of Louis.* It can be felt as a slight transverse ridge across the sternum about 3·0 cm (1⅜ in) below the floor of the sternal notch, and its position can be confirmed by finding, a little laterally and at the same level, the second costal cartilage which articulates with the sternum at this level. In quiet respiration the sternal angle lies at the level of the disc between T4 and T5. When the angle is difficult to find, palpation is best carried out using a circular motion of the fingers over its anticipated position (*Plate* 3).

The position of the anterior end of the second rib and its costal cartilage can be traced out laterally from the junction of the cartilage with the sternum at the sternal angle. The *first intercostal space* will be felt immediately above it and just below the medial part of the clavicle. Once the position of the second rib and its costal cartilage have been established, recognition of other ribs and the counting of intercostal spaces is straightforward. The *fourth intercostal space* is usually indicated by the position of the nipple in the male. In the female the nipple is unreliable for this purpose. The position of the *fifth rib* is indicated by the lower edge of the *pectoralis major* muscle and by the line where the breast joins the chest wall (*Plate* 3).

The *xiphoid process* is easily found in any subject. Its shape varies considerably and it may be found to be straight, bifid, perforated or less commonly deviated to either side or even slightly protruding. In most subjects it is slightly springy. Its junction with the body of the sternum is at the level of the disc between T9 and T10, in quiet respiration. The lower intercostal spaces can be identified and enumerated easily. Palpation to find the level of the lowest point of the *lower costal margin* should employ the heel of the hand in order to avoid the mildly convulsive effect which may be initiated by use of the fingertips for this purpose in some subjects. The

level of the lowest part of the lower costal margin corresponds
to that of the body of the 3rd lumbar vertebra (*Plate* 4).

POSTERIOR ASPECT
The spinous processes of the thoracic vertebrae can be made
out as a series of firm projections in the midline posteriorly,
but there is difficulty in immediate precise identification of
individual processes. When the subject leans forward there is
increased prominence of the processes and counting becomes
easier. Identification can be made quite confidently by counting downwards once the 7th cervical vertebral process has been
recognized. It will be recalled that this is the first recognizable
midline posterior bony prominence in the lower part of the
posterior aspect of the neck, and that the 1st thoracic vertebral
spinous process is almost as prominent in many subjects.

The *inferior scapular angles* are quite prominent in most
subjects and hardly require palpation for recognition. The
angles usually lie at the level of the 9th thoracic vertebral body
and generally lie over part of the 8th rib. This assumes an
average subject in the conventional anatomical position but
individual variations can be quite marked and vary with
posture. The *vertebral borders* of the *scapulae* seen in the
relaxed subject parallel to the spine, incline away sharply when
the arms are raised and the *angles* of the *scapulae* move in an
arc to the sides. The *spine* of the *scapula* can be traced out
visually in thin subjects and on many well covered ones
requires only light palpation to reveal its position. The
acromion is easily felt and the prominent *acromion angle* at
the junction of the posterior and lateral parts of the acromion
can be felt as a quite distinct point (*Plate* 5).

The *coracoid process,* used as a radiographic centring point
for the general anteroposterior projection of the shoulder can
be found near the shoulder joint just below the clavicle if firm
palpation is used. This is ill-advised when examining a patient
with a shoulder injury and it is prudent to gain reasonable
familiarity with its likely position on normal subjects to
facilitate easy recognition in more difficult clinical situations.

Chapter 6

The Arm

It is difficult to make out the upper parts of the humerus at the shoulder joint due to muscle coverage. Pressure over the rounded lateral part of the shoulder provides only a dull impression of the *greater tuberosity* of the *humerus* which lies under it (*Plates* 1 and 5). Upward pressure into the *axilla,* the deep hollow below the arm where it joins the thorax, will detect, but usually not clearly, part of the *head* of the *humerus* if the arm is actively rotated during palpation. The upper parts of the humerus are not easily felt but careful exploration of the lateral part of the axilla will locate part of the humeral shaft and in most subjects it is possible to make out the *surgical neck* of the *humerus* with a little care. It becomes easier to palpate the humeral shaft below the deltoid muscle.

REGION OF THE ELBOW

The *supracondylar ridges* and the *medial* and *lateral epicondyles* can be readily found. The medial ridge is usually easier to trace out. The groove for the ulnar nerve can be felt on the back of the medial epicondyle and the nerve made to roll within it by suitable pressure. The *olecranon process* of the *ulna* will be recognized as the very obvious point of the elbow. It is less easy to find the *radial head* which can best be felt from behind the elbow and lateral to the olecranon process when the arm is extended. Its position can be verified by feeling it roll at the superior radio-ulnar joint when the wrist is rotated (*Fig.* 10). It is not possible to palpate the elbow joint itself but the position of the general transverse line of the joint can be indicated by a line drawn transversely

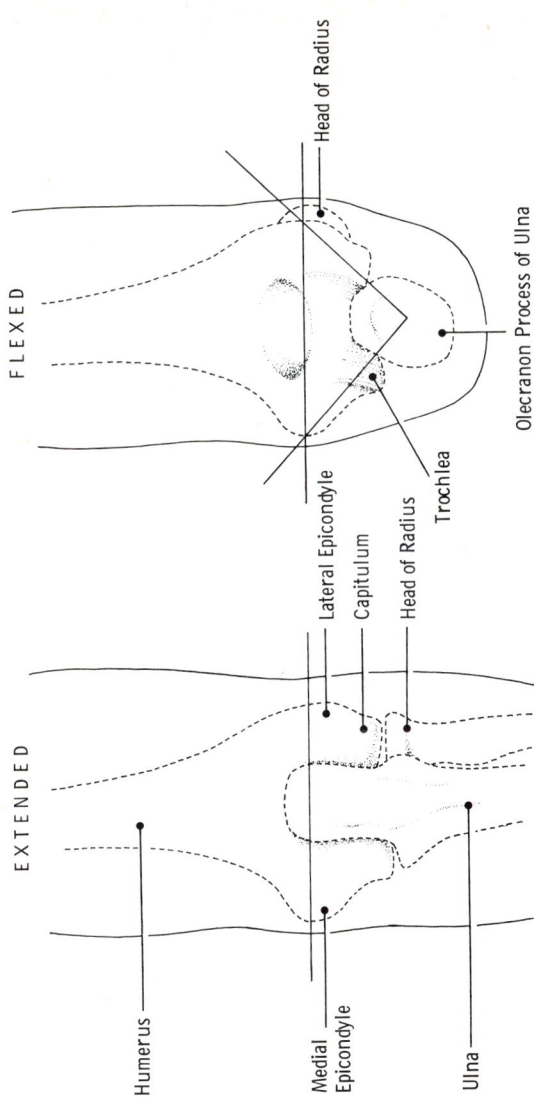

Fig. 10. Bony landmarks of elbow.

across the elbow region 2·5 cm (1 in) below and parallel to a line joining the epicondyles of the humerus.

The *olecranon* and the *medial* and *lateral epicondyles* lie on a straight line when the elbow is extended, with the *olecranon* midway between the *epicondyles*. They form an equilateral triangle when the elbow is flexed to a right angle (*Fig.* 10).

Whereas it is always possible to feel some part of the *ulna* over its whole length, the *radius* is only intermittently palpable at its upper end. At its lower end its termination can be felt as a well-defined transverse ridge anteriorly about 2·5 cm (1 in) above the thenar eminence. The tip of the *radial styloid process* can be found in the proximal part of the *anatomical snuff box* at the lateral side of the wrist (*Fig.* 11 and *Plate* 6). The *lower end* of the *radius* can be felt posteriorly by a finger making upward and forward pressure from behind the wrist. The *pisiform* can be recognized on the anterior aspect of the wrist as the bony prominence at the *hypothenar eminence.* It is easily felt on the medial side of the wrist and the direction of the *flexor carpi ulnaris* tendon is a further guide to its position (*Fig.* 11). On the anterior aspect of the wrist the *tubercle* of the *scaphoid* can be made out about two finger spaces laterally from a finger placed over the *pisiform* bone. It is immediately above the thenar eminence. The *tubercle* of the *trapezium* can be felt just distal to the scaphoid tubercle but it is not easily recognized and requires patient exploration to verify its position since it is only dully perceived. Palpation of the floor and distal part of the anatomical snuff box will indicate the positions of part of the *scaphoid* and the *trapezium.*

The position of the *hook of the hamate* can be found if the index finger is placed over the pisiform and deep pressure is then applied by the middle forefinger placed fairly close to it along a line between the pisiform and the centre of the palm (*Fig.* 11).

The *ulnar styloid process* can be felt on the back of the wrist when the hand is *supinated.*

On the back of the hand it is possible to identify the bases

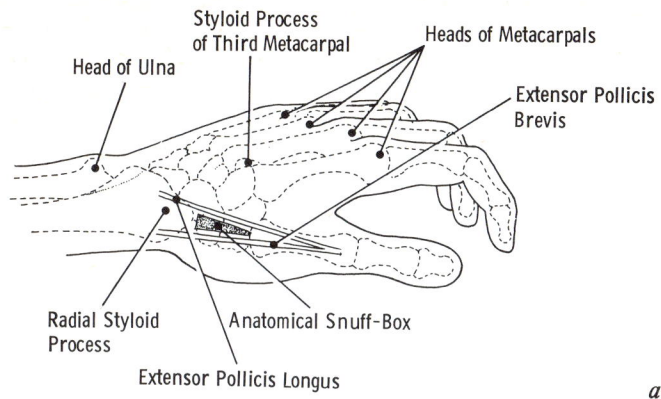

a

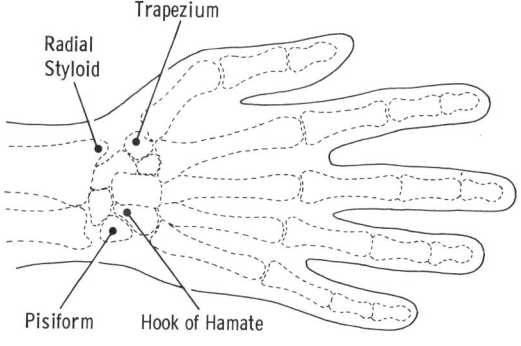

b

Fig. 11. Bony landmarks of (*a*) wrist; (*b*) hand.

of the *first, third* and *fifth metacarpals* and to find the styloid process of the third metacarpal.

The *heads of the metacarpals* can be examined easily when the fist is clenched and the knuckles become prominent. It is tempting to mistake a line drawn across the webs of the fingers on the palmar aspect of the hand as an indication of the position of the metacarpophalangeal joints which in fact lie about 2·0 cm ($\frac{3}{4}$ in) proximal to them. Examination of the lateral aspect of the hand marking the position of the knuckles will confirm this. Of the creases overlying the approximate region of each interphalangeal joint on the palmar aspect of the hand, the most distal in each case should be taken as indicating the position of the joint.

Chapter 7

The lumbar and pelvic regions

Little of the lumbar vertebrae can be palpated other than the spinous processes which are best found well separated when the subject bends forward. In the erect position they are not easily distinguished. The level of the lower costal margin may be taken as an approximate guide to the level of the *3rd lumbar vertebral body* but this is liable to considerable variation due to subject type and particularly in the elderly. It should be noted that the position of the spinous process of a lumbar vertebra lies approximately at the level of the lower border of its vertebral body. The *4th lumbar spinous process* lies at the level of the highest part of the iliac crest.

The *iliac crest* is palpable over its entire length and is more prominent in subjects whose musculature is weak or wasted. The position of the *posterior superior iliac spine* can be recognized visually by the dimpling effect it produces just above the buttocks and about two finger spaces from the midline. A finger pressed into the dimple, which can be recognized on all subjects will locate the firm resistance of the posterior superior iliac spine in its floor (*Plate* 7). It is a reliable guide to the position of the middle of the *sacro-iliac joint* and also lies at the level of the *2nd sacral spine.* The tip of the *coccyx* is accessible to careful palpation and needs to be very accurately located for radiographic centring when coned lateral projection is undertaken if misalignment in the small area beam is to be avoided. The *posterior sacral surface,* being superficial, is readily explored. The upper limit of the *gluteal cleft* which separates the buttocks in the midline reaches close to the level of the 3rd sacral segment.

The *ischial tuberosities* can be palpated on deep pressure at

33

the line delineating the lower fold of the buttocks. The student will already be aware of their positions if seated for any considerable length of time on a hard surface.

The *anterior superior iliac spine* is readily found in any subject and becomes particularly prominent when seated. When standing it is at the same level as the *posterior superior iliac spine* (*Plate* 7). It is important as a landmark and in finding radiographic centring points for a variety of examinations in the pelvic region. The *tubercle* of the *iliac crest* is found 6 cm (2⅜ in) above and behind the anterior superior iliac spine and is the most lateral part of the iliac crest. It is used as a reference point from which the *transtubercular plane* and *line* are produced for abdominal topographical description. The upper border of the *pubic bone* at the *symphysis pubis,* the junction of one side with the other, is of equal radiographic significance as a landmark and is readily located using the edge of the hand (*Plate* 4). The *pubic tubercle,* found easily in the male about 2·0 cm (¾ in) from the midline along the upper border of the pubic bone is less readily found in the female since it is less developed. Its position can be found by tracing downwards from the anterior superior iliac spine along the *inguinal ligament* which can be felt as a taut cordlike structure terminating at the pubic tubercle. Furthermore, the *tendon* of the *adductor longus* muscle which is quite easily recognized can be traced to its origin immediately below and medial to the tubercle (*Plate* 8).

The *pubic arch* formed by the divergent rami of the pubis on each side is palpable through the scrotum from below in the male. The rami are more widely divergent anteriorly and easily found in the female.

Chapter 8

The femoral region and leg

The *greater trochanter* of the *femur* can be felt in front of the large shallow depression close to the lateral gluteal region. It is easy to palpate in the standing subject when weight is taken on the opposite leg and it is then possible to feel its upper border which is at the level of the centre of the hip joint and the upper border of the symphysis pubis. The *lesser trochanter* can be palpated, though with some difficulty on deep upward pressure to the medial aspect of the upper thigh. The *head of the femur* cannot be felt clearly except when it is in movement, and even then not particularly well. Its surface projection on the anterior aspect is easily delineated by taking a line between the *anterior superior iliac spine* and the upper border of the *symphysis pubis,* bisecting it at right angles and taking a point 2·5 cm (1 in) along the bisecting line. This will overlie the *femoral head (Fig.* 12). Pressure using a finger over this point will detect the pulsation of the *femoral artery* confirming the location since the artery is palpable where it crossed the femoral head. The *femoral neck* cannot be felt, but its approximate alignment from the anterior aspect can be estimated by taking a line from the position of the femoral head to the lowest part of the greater trochanter. The *femoral shaft* is heavily muscle covered and mostly inaccessible to palpation. Its general alignment from the anterior aspect may be indicated by a line drawn from a point about 2·5 cm (1 in) medial to the most lateral part of the *greater trochanter* to the *apex* of the *patella (Plate* 8).

REGION OF THE KNEE
The *adductor tubercle* can be found most readily in the seated subject by following with the fingers the lower edge of the

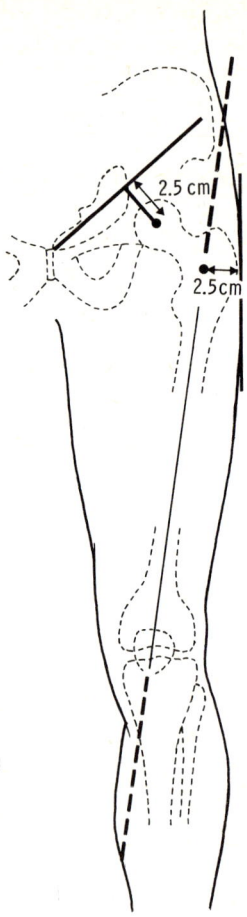

Fig. 12. Surface markings of femoral head.

vastus medialis muscle on the medial aspect of the thigh. A little pressure with the fingertips will locate the tendon of the *adductor magnus* muscle which terminates in the *adductor tubercle,* which can now be recognized proximal to the medial femoral condyle. The *medial condyle* of the *femur* is very prominent, indeed visibly so in thin subjects, medial to the ligamentum patellae and its margin may be followed easily from there. The *lateral condyle* of the *femur* can also be found easily and traced round by starting in the other depression just lateral to the ligamentum patellae but it is helpful in this instance to keep the musculature around the knee well relaxed. There is normally no difficulty in identifying the interval between the femoral condyles and the tibia anteriorly by pressure to either side of the ligamentum patellae. There is greater difficulty in finding the anterior edges of the medial and lateral *semilunar cartilages* which are elusive in many subjects although it is possible to make them out rather indistinctly in some. The *patella* shows its position easily in thin subjects and is very easily found. When the leg is relaxed the *patella* may be displaced to either side by light sustained pressure and moved up and down on being lightly gripped. When the leg is extended its apex lies about 2·5 cm (1 in) above the anterior edge of the tibial table. The apex is an important landmark from which several radiographic centring points are measured (*Plate* 9 and *Fig.* 13). The anterior edge of the *'tibial table'* can be recognized when the fingers are pushed downwards towards it from the level of the patella when the knee is bent. Much of the upper end of the tibia can be felt anteriorly, laterally and medially but is not palpable posteriorly. The rounded protuberance below it on the lateral aspect of the knee recognized by palm pressure against the region is the *head* of the *fibula.* The tendon of the *long head* of the *biceps femoris,* the very prominent tendon visible on the lateral aspect of the knee, is inserted into it and acts as a further guide to its position. It is possible to follow the *shaft* of the *fibula* for only a very short distance below the head as it becomes obscured by overlying muscle. The *lateral surface* of

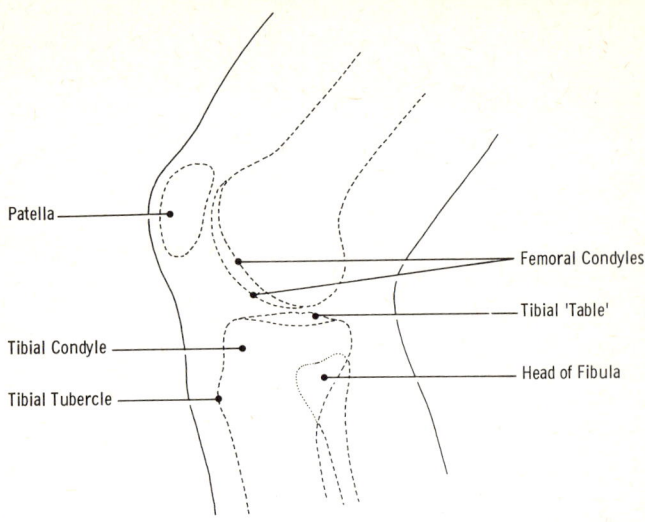

Patella

Femoral Condyles

Tibial 'Table'

Tibial Condyle

Head of Fibula

Tibial Tubercle

Fig. 13. Bony landmarks of knee.

the *tibial shaft* is not accessible to palpation but quite the reverse is true of the *anterior border* and the *medial surface* which are subcutaneous. The *anterior border* with its visible *sinuous line* is so prominent as to have no need of palpation for recognition. The whole of the *medial surface* can be felt.

When in the kneeling position the weight of the body is taken on the anterior part of the *tibial tubercle* just above the *sinuous line* of the anterior tibial border (*Plate* 9).

REGION OF THE ANKLE AND FOOT

The lower part of the fibula becomes distinctly palpable about 15 cm (6 in) above the lateral malleolus which extends downwards a little below the level of the medial malleolus. Firm pressure with a fingertip upwards and forwards from behind the lowest part of the lateral malleolus will detect the position of the groove for the peroneal tendons.

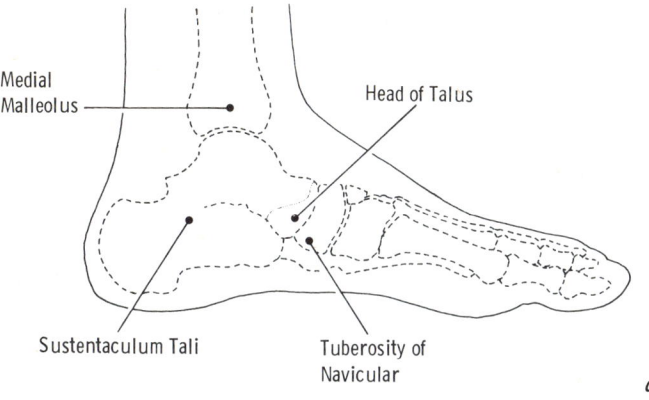

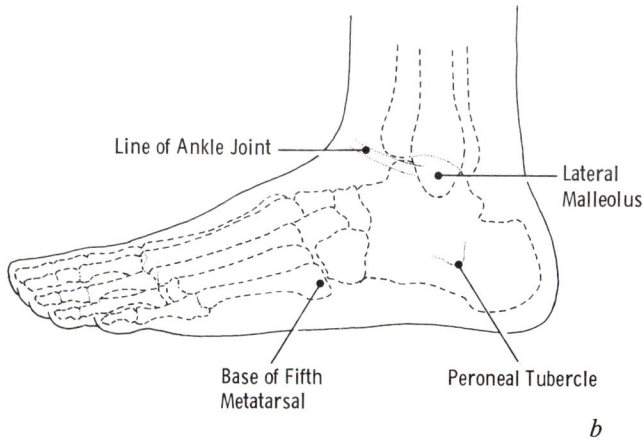

Fig. 14. (*a*) Medial aspect of foot; (*b*) Lateral aspect of foot.

Exploration of the lower part of the *anterior aspect* of the *tibia* is impeded by tendons crossing it but to either side of these extensor tendons, the line of the ankle joint is accessible to palpation bordered above by the lower tibial margin. When the foot is extended fully and inverted (turned so that the sole faces as far medially as possible) the *head* of the *talus* becomes evident and is easily felt about 2·5 cm (1 in) in front of the ankle joint. A fingertip pressing firmly medially just below and anterior to the lateral malleolus will locate the *neck* of the *talus*. The *sustentaculum tali* can be felt as a firm ridge about 2·5 cm (1 in) below the medial malleolus and the *talocalcaneal* joint lies immediately above it. All of the *lateral surface* of the *calcaneus* is accessible to palpation and the *peroneal tubercle* is identifiable without difficulty in most subjects. The posterior part of the calcaneus carries two tubercles, medial and lateral, which are sufficiently prominent to be palpable on deep pressure posteriorly from the plantar aspect of the heel. The *tuberosity* of the *navicular bone* can be detected by a finger stroked forwards along the medial aspect of the foot, followed as the finger continues forward by the *base* and then the *head* of the *first metatarsal*. A similar approach to the lateral edge of the foot will locate the *base* and the *head* of the *fifth metatarsal* when palpation begins along the edge of the foot from below the lateral malleolus (*Fig.* 14).

The position of the *metatarsophalangeal joints* lies about 2·5 cm (1 in) behind the webs on the toes.

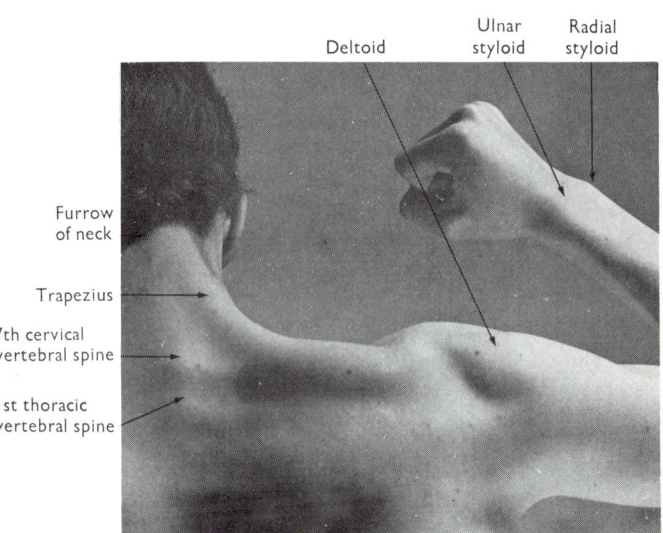

Plate 1. Posterior view of neck and shoulder.

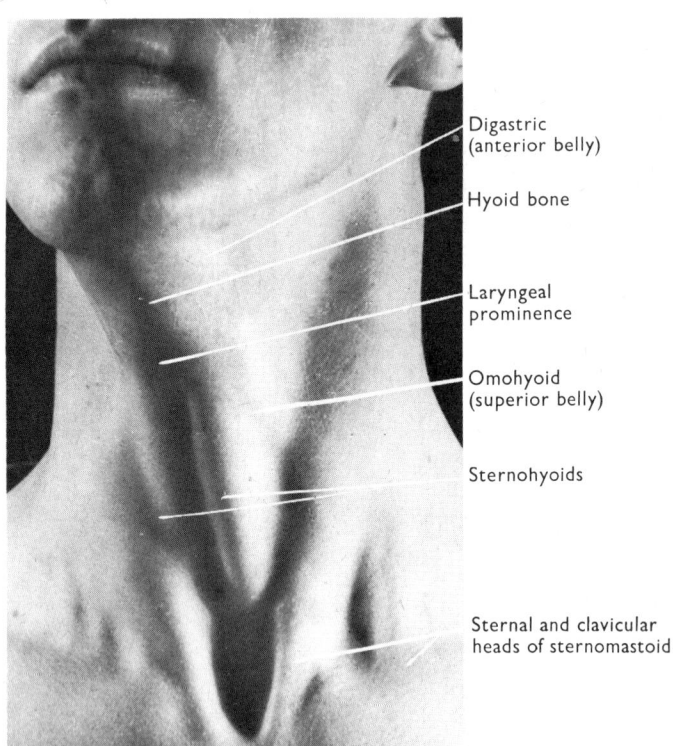

Digastric
(anterior belly)

Hyoid bone

Laryngeal
prominence

Omohyoid
(superior belly)

Sternohyoids

Sternal and clavicular
heads of sternomastoid

Plate 2. Anterior view of chin and neck, chin raised and muscles set.
*(Reproduced by permission of Faber & Faber Ltd from 'Living
Anatomy' by Professor R. D. Lockhart.)*

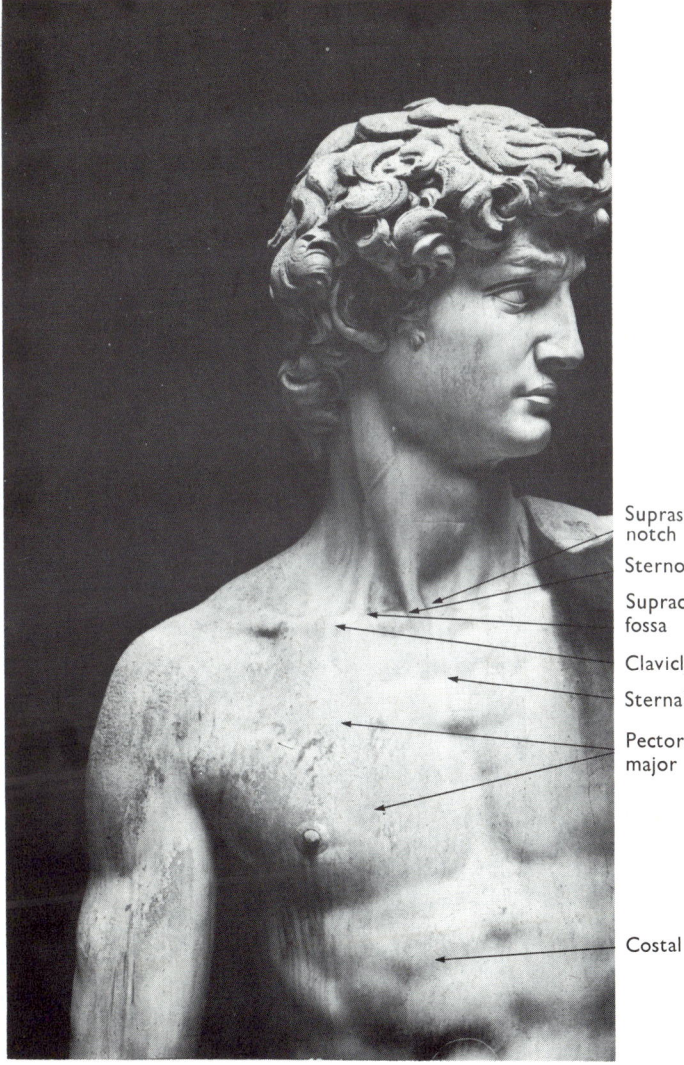

Suprasternal
notch

Sternomastoid

Supraclavicular
fossa

Clavicle

Sternal angle

Pectoralis
major

Costal margin

Plate 3. Anterior view of thorax. *(Reproduced by permission of the Mansell Collection, London: Print from Fratelli Alinari, Florence (Michaelangelo's David).)*

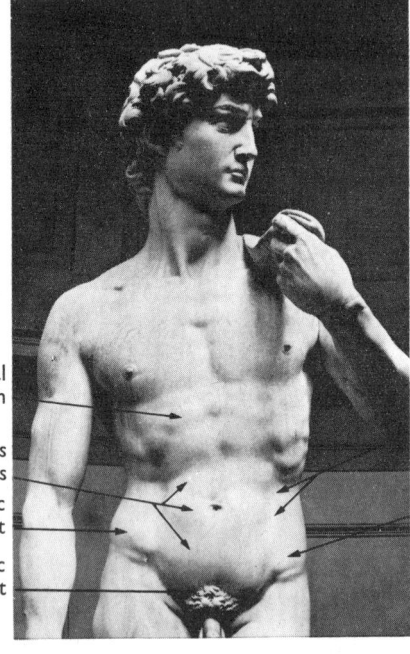

Costal margin

Rectus abdominis

Iliac crest

Pubic crest

Linea semilunaris

Anterior superior iliac spine

Plate 4. Anterior view of abdomen. *(Reproduced by permission of the Mansell Collection, London: Print from Fratelli Alinari, Florence (Michaelangelo's David).)*

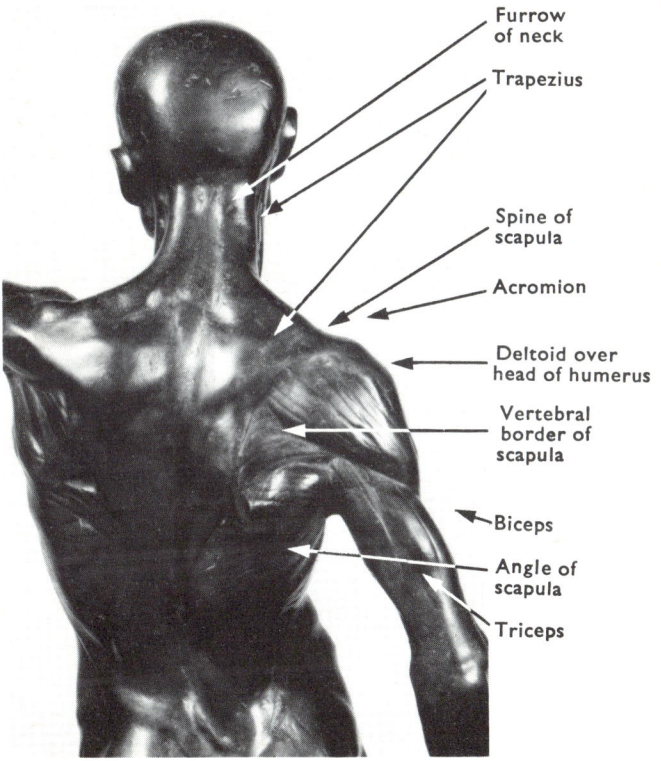

Furrow
of neck

Trapezius

Spine of
scapula

Acromion

Deltoid over
head of humerus

Vertebral
border of
scapula

Biceps

Angle of
scapula

Triceps

Plate 5. Shoulder region, posterior view. *(Crown Copyright. Victoria and Albert Museum.)*

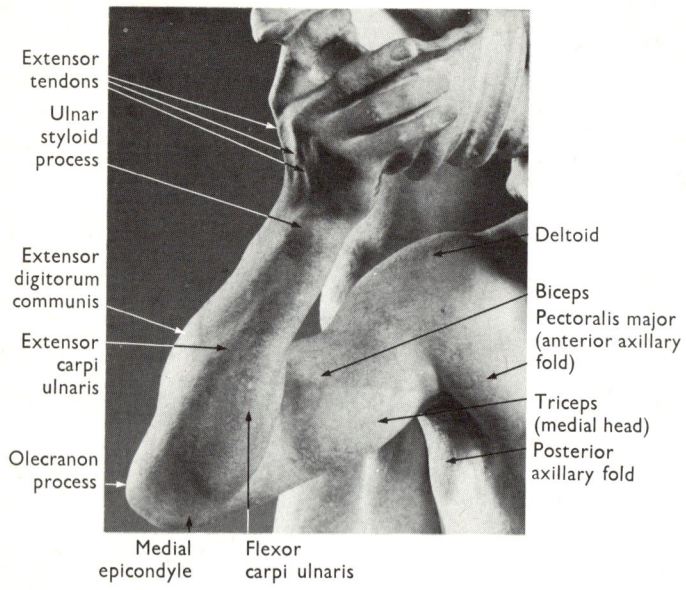

Extensor
tendons

Ulnar
styloid
process

Extensor
digitorum
communis

Extensor
carpi
ulnaris

Olecranon
process

Medial
epicondyle

Flexor
carpi ulnaris

Deltoid

Biceps

Pectoralis major
(anterior axillary
fold)

Triceps
(medial head)

Posterior
axillary fold

Plate 6. Forearm and hand. *(Crown Copyright. Victoria and Albert Museum.)*

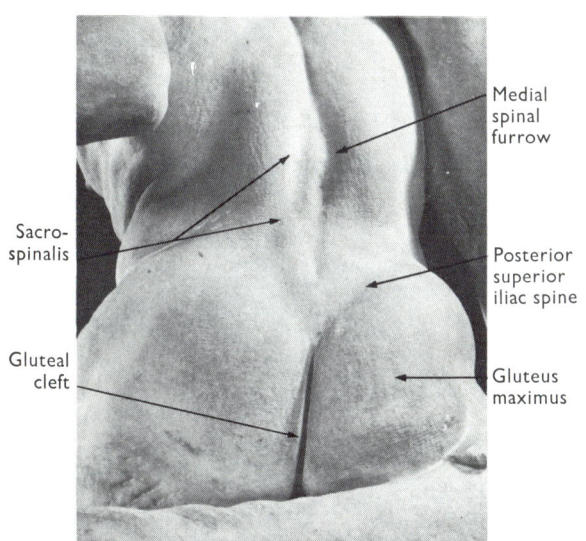

Medial
spinal
furrow

Sacro-
spinalis

Posterior
superior
iliac spine

Gluteal
cleft

Gluteus
maximus

Plate 7. Lumbar spine and trunk. *(Crown Copyright. Victoria and Albert Museum.)*

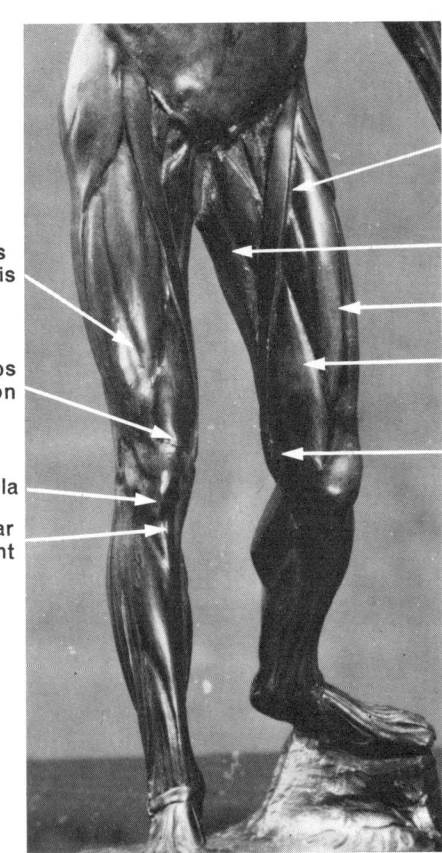

Sartorius

Adductor
muscles

Rectus
femoris

Vastus
medialis

Medial
femoral
condyle

Vastus
lateralis

Quadriceps
tendon

Patella

Patellar
ligament

Plate 8. Thigh, anterior view. *(Crown Copyright. Victoria and Albert Museum.)*

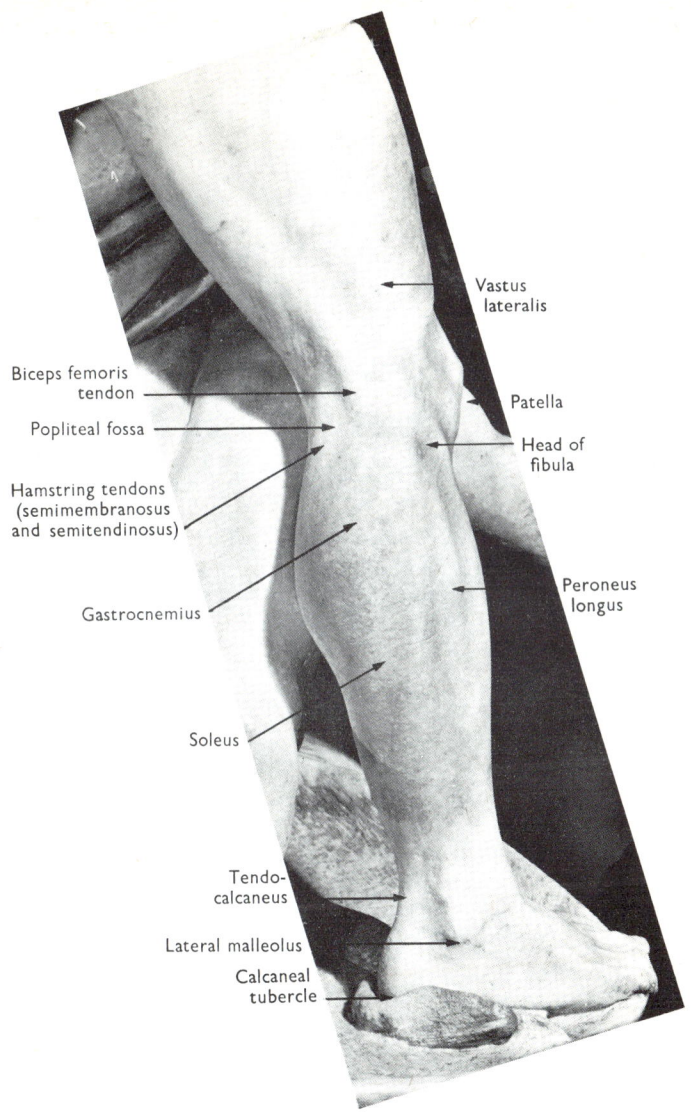

Vastus
lateralis

Biceps femoris
tendon

Patella

Popliteal fossa

Head of
fibula

Hamstring tendons
(semimembranosus
and semitendinosus)

Peroneus
longus

Gastrocnemius

Soleus

Tendo-
calcaneus

Lateral malleolus

Calcaneal
tubercle

Plate 9. Lower leg and calf. *(Crown Copyright. Victoria and Albert Museum.)*

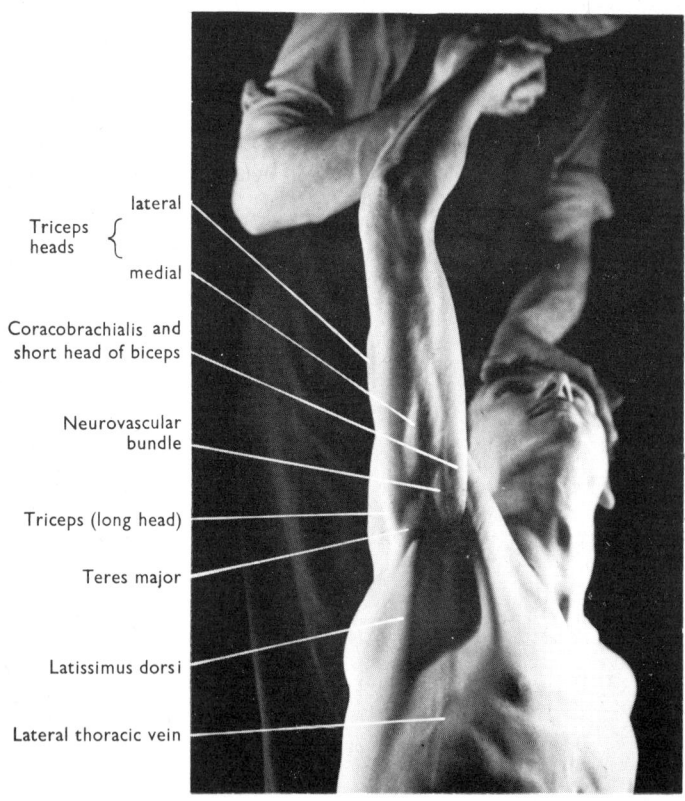

lateral
Triceps heads {
medial

Coracobrachialis and
short head of biceps

Neurovascular
bundle

Triceps (long head)

Teres major

Latissimus dorsi

Lateral thoracic vein

Plate 10. Axilla. Triceps extending elbow against resistance. Note biceps running into axilla posterior to pectoralis major, and the position of the neurovascular bundle. *(Reproduced by permission of Faber & Faber Ltd from 'Living Anatomy' by Professor R. D. Lockhart.)*

Part 2

Surface anatomy of the soft tissues

Having studied the bony landmarks of the skeleton in Part 1, the second part of the book describes the surface markings of the soft tissues, dealing with visible structures, muscles, underlying organs and vessels.

Chapter 9

The head and neck

The soft-tissue structures of the head and neck which include the eye, nose, ear and mouth, can be studied by direct observation.

THE EYE

The space between the eyelids is termed the *palpebral fissure* with the *angles* of the *eye* or medial and lateral canthi forming its ends (*Fig.* 15). When the eyelids are separated the surface of the eyeball may be seen to consist of a bluish-white portion, the *sclera,* into which is set the transparent *cornea* which forms a slight anterior bulge from the otherwise spherical surface. An annular pigmented structure with faint radial markings is seen through the cornea. This is the *iris* which contracts in strong light conditions. Those parts of the eye region most commonly used as landmarks are the *pupil,* the aperture within the iris, and the *canthi,* though it is mainly the *lateral canthus* which is commonly used. Towards the medial ends of the eyelids the eyelashes disappear and a small papilla is seen on both upper and lower lids, each carrying a *punctum lacrimale* (*Fig.* 15) which drains tears which form at the *lacrimal lake.* The *puncta lacrimalia* are the tiny orifices of the upper and lower *lacrimal canaliculi.* It is these which must be dilated and then entered by a *lacrimal probe* and *cannula* to enable the necessary injection of radiopaque contrast medium to be given to demonstrate the patency or otherwise of the *lacrimal ducts* during the examination called *dacryocystography.* The lacrimal lake forms between the surface of the eyeball and the small reddish *lacrimal caruncle* just inside the medial canthus of the eye (*Figs.* 7 and 15). If the eyelids are turned back, a

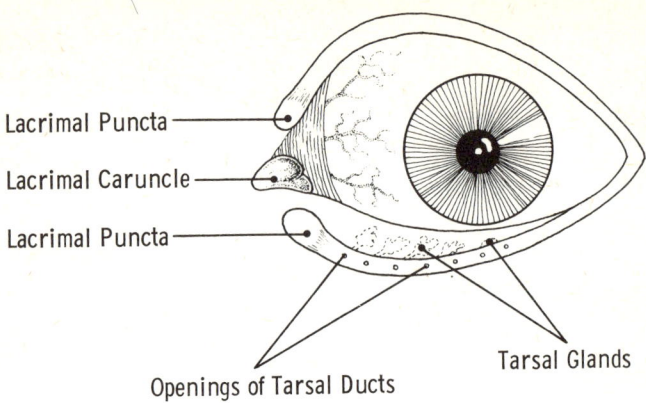

Fig. 15. Eye and eyelids.

plate of dense tissue in each lid, called the *tarsus,* makes it possible for the lid to remain in that position, especially the upper lid, without further assistance. When this is done, or even if the lids are just a little everted the *tarsal glands* may be seen inside the lid as a series of fine yellowish lines radiating outwards to the edge of the lid. The orifices of the ducts, along the edge of the lid are very fine and much less readily seen than most anatomical illustrations would suggest (*Fig.* 15).

THE NOSE

The nose varies individually in size and shape and although its tip is used as a radiographic centring point in dental work this should not be taken to imply anything more than a very general constancy of relationship to other structures. The *ala* of the nose, that is the curved portion at the side of each nostril where it joins the face, is used as a clearly visible landmark for drawing out various lines as indicators for the positions of structures such as *Stensen's duct* and for some dental radiographic positioning lines (*Figs.* 4 and 5).

Inspection of the nostrils shows them to be hair-lined within their terminal portions, bounded superiorly by a lateral

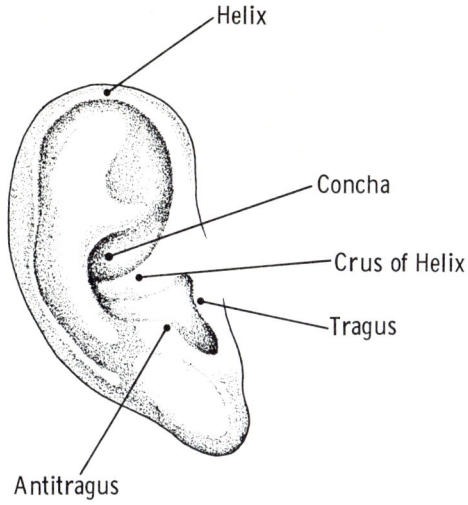

Fig. 16. External ear.

ridge termed the *limen nasi*. If the nostrils are dilated and the tip of the nose pushed back, some parts of the nasal cavities can be seen by the aid of a suitable small electric torch. The *inferior nasal concha* is seen as a pink projection from the side of the nostril and above it the *middle nasal concha* can be made out rather lighter in colour.

THE EAR
The external ear is composed of two parts, the *external auditory meatus* and the *auricle*. The auricle varies considerably in shape and size between individuals but exhibits certain constant features. Immediately in front of the external auditory meatus there is a small springy rearward-pointing flap called the *tragus*. It is prominent, readily seen and used as a visual landmark. Just above the lobe of the ear which is fleshy and pendulous to a variable degree is the *antitragus* which generally resembles the tragus but points upwards. The large

flattened area behind the meatus is termed the *concha* and is divided into upper and lower parts by the *crus* of the *helix*. The concha is bounded superiorly and posteriorly by the *antihelix* which divides superiorly into an *upper* and *lower crus* with the *triangular fossa* between. A small tubercle may be noted on the posterior part of the helix and it is thought that this corresponds to the point of the ear in some higher animals (*Fig.* 16). A very limited degree of voluntary movement of the auricle can be achieved by some individuals. The angle made by the auricle against the side of the head is usually around 30°, an angle to which the auricle rapidly returns even after prolonged displacement.

The *external auditory meatus* leads from the concha to the middle ear, is partly cartilaginous and lined with skin and a variable amount of hair externally. It can be inspected if the auricle is pulled upwards and forwards to straighten its normal curvature but an aural speculum is required for examination of its whole length.

THE MOUTH

The *mouth* is bounded by the lips anteriorly and consists of the vestibule and the mouth cavity proper. These are separated by the teeth and gums. The lips consist of skin externally, lined with mucous membranes internally, with the *orbicularis oris muscle* between (*see below*). The lips bound the mouth orifice and meet laterally at the angles of the mouth.

MUSCLES OF HEAD AND NECK

Under the skin, the vault of the skull is covered by a thin aponeurosis, consisting of a sheet of white fibrous tissue. This connects the anterior and posterior parts of the *occipito-frontalis* muscle. The muscle is attached posteriorly along the superior nuchal line of the occipital bone. It raises the eyebrows and wrinkles the forehead.

Other facial muscles are:

Levator palpebrae superioris, originating from the posterior part of the orbital cavity and inserted into the tarsal plate of the upper eyelid. It raises the eyelid.

Orbicularis oculi, surrounds the eye, and closes it.

Orbicularis oris, surrounds the mouth, and closes it.

In the cheeks is situated the *buccinator* muscle, consisting of a flat sheet of muscle on either side of the oral cavity. It draws in the cheeks. The floor of the mouth is formed by the *mylohyoid* and *geniohyoid* muscles, which originate from the inner surface of the body of the mandible and symphysis menti, and are inserted into the hyoid bone.

Below the hyoid, the *thyrohyoid* muscle connects the hyoid to the thyroid cartilage, and from thence the *sternothyroid* muscle connects the thyroid cartilage to the sternum and clavicle, covering the larynx and trachea. Over both of these is the *sternohyoid* muscle, originating from the sternum and clavicle and inserted into the lower border of the hyoid bone.

The *cricothyroid* membrane fills the gap between the thyroid and cricoid cartilages (*Fig.* 9).

A small slim muscle, the *omohyoid,* can often be seen below the skin, extending from the hyoid down towards the clavicle and then under the sternomastoid muscle, backwards towards the scapula (*Plate* 2).

The *temporalis muscle* occupies the temporal fossa of the skull, with a tendon passing under the zygomatic arch to be inserted into the coronoid process and anterior border of the mandibular ramus. It can be felt when the teeth are clenched.

The *masseter muscle* originates from the zygomatic arch and is inserted into the lateral surface of the ramus and angle of the mandible. It overlies the ramus.

The *sternomastoid* muscle can be seen crossing the neck diagonally from the upper border of the manubrium sterni and medial end of the clavicle, to be inserted into the mastoid process of the skull. It is most evident when the head is turned to the opposite side (*Plates* 2 and 3).

On either side of the back of the neck, can be seen the *semispinalis capitis* muscles with a groove between them, in the midline. This line represents the line of the ligamentum nuchae, connecting the cervical spinous processes to the occipital protuberance of the skull. It extends down as far as the prominent 7th cervical vertebra. The *trapezius muscle* covers the side and back of the neck and upper posterior thorax, originating from the cervical and thoracic spinous processes and inserted into the adjacent borders of the spine of the scapula, and the clavicle (*Plate* 1). The sternomastoid muscle divides the neck into *anterior* and *posterior triangles* (*Plate* 3).

The *anterior triangle* is bounded posteriorly by the anterior border of the sternomastoid muscle, above by the lower margin of the body of the mandible and anteriorly by the median plane.

The *posterior triangle* is bounded anteriorly by the posterior border of the sternomastoid muscle, below by the middle third of the clavicle and posteriorly by the trapezius muscle.

The hollow in its lower part, immediately above the clavicle, is the *supraclavicular fossa* (*Plate* 2) through which runs the subclavian artery, which can be felt pulsating, on deep pressure.

Below the middle third of the clavicles is the hollow of the *infraclavicular fossa.*

Between the two sternomastoid muscles, immediately above the upper margin of the manubrium sterni, is the *suprasternal notch,* or fossa, situated at the level of the 2nd thoracic vertebra (*Plate* 3).

SALIVARY GLANDS

THE PAROTID GLAND

The parotid gland occupies a depression behind the ramus of the mandible, extending forwards onto the masseter muscle (*see below*), overlying the angle of the mandible. It is roughly pyramidal in shape, with the apex downward. Below, it extends 2 cm (¾ in) below the angle of the mandible.

Surface markings can be represented as follows:

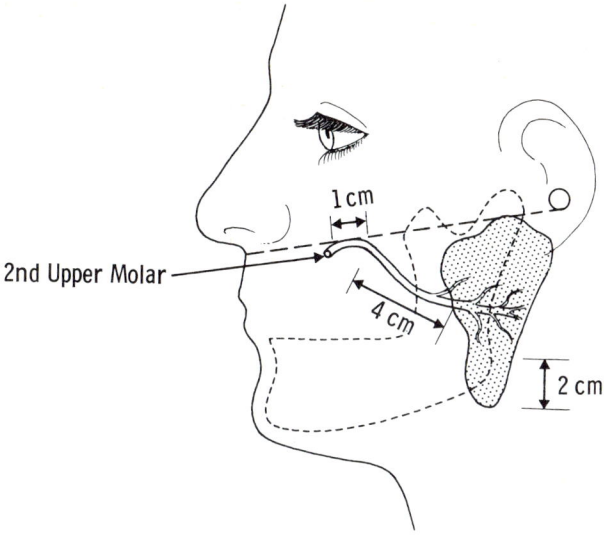

Fig. 17. Parotid gland and duct.

Anterior Border: A line downwards and forwards from the upper border of the mandibular condyle to a point just above the middle of the masseter muscle, and then downwards and backwards to a point 2 cm ($\frac{3}{4}$ in) below and behind the angle of the mandible.

Upper Border: A curved line concave upwards and backwards from the upper border of the mandibular condyle across the lobule of the auricle to the mastoid process.

Posterior Border: A straight line joining the ends of the anterior and upper borders.

The *parotid duct* is about 5 cm (2 in) long and runs upwards and forwards from a point 2 cm ($\frac{3}{4}$ in) above the angle of the mandible near the centre of the parotid gland, to a point 1 cm ($\frac{3}{8}$ in) behind the junction of the middle and anterior thirds of a line from the external auditory meatus to the midpoint between the ala of the nose and upper lip margin (*Fig.* 17).

(Previous texts have described it as lying on the middle third of this line, but a glance at a parotid sialogram will show that this is incorrect.)

Here it loops inward around the masseter muscle and penetrates the buccinator, opening into the mouth on the inner surface of the cheek opposite the second upper molar tooth.

THE SUBMANDIBULAR GLAND

The submandibular gland is situated medially to the angle of the mandible, in the submandibular fossae. Its duct (5 cm (2 in) long) runs forward in the floor of the mouth, from the gland to the orifice situated close to the frenulum of the tongue, near the midline, about 2 cm ($\frac{3}{4}$ in) behind the point of the chin.

THE SUBLINGUAL GLANDS

The *sublingual glands* lie in the floor of the mouth anteriorly, lateral to the submandibular ducts, on either side of the frenulum of the tongue (*Fig.* 18).

THE LARYNX

The *larynx* is situated behind the thyroid and cricoid cartilages, at the upper end of the trachea. These cartilages can be felt in the midline of the neck, below the *hyoid* bone (situated at the base of the tongue). The upper border of the *thyroid cartilage* forms the prominent 'Adam's Apple' (opposite C4). This is more prominent in men, after puberty, owing to the larger size of the adult male larynx, and is used as a radiographic centring point for the larynx (*see Fig.* 9).

Below the thyroid cartilage is the signet-ring-shaped *cricoid cartilage,* which can be felt about 2 cm ($\frac{3}{4}$ in) above the upper border of the manubrium sterni (opposite C6) forming the uppermost ring of the trachea (*Plate* 2).

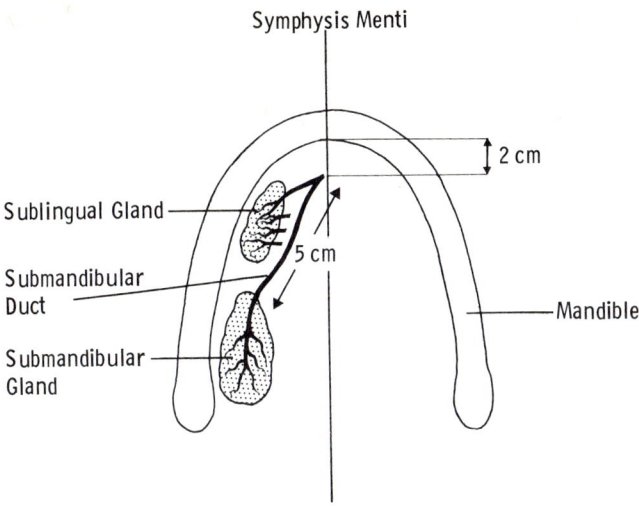

Fig. 18. Submandibular and sublingual glands and ducts, interior view.

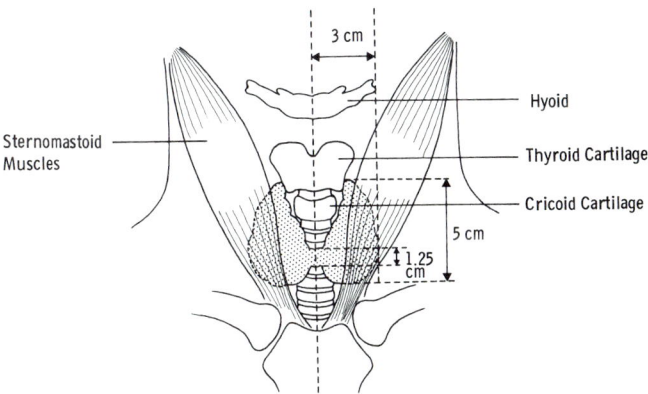

Fig. 19. Thyroid gland.

THE THYROID

The *thyroid gland* has two lobes, joined by the isthmus, situated on either side of the trachea and larynx. Each lobe is about 5 cm (2 in) long and 3 cm (1¼ in) wide. They extend downwards from the middle of the thyroid cartilage and almost meet in the midline anteriorly (*Fig.* 19). The isthmus lies in front of the trachea, 2 cm (¾ in) below the cricoid cartilage, overlying the 3rd and 4th rings of the trachea. It is about 1·25 cm (½ in) deep. When enlarged the thyroid may extend down to, or sometimes behind the clavicles and manubrium of the sternum.

VESSELS

The *common carotid artery* is situated behind the anterior border of the sternomastoid muscle, along a line from the sternoclavicular joint to the upper border of the thyroid cartilage (opposite C4) (*Fig.* 20).

At the level of the upper border of the thyroid cartilage, the common carotid artery divides into *external and internal carotid arteries* (at the level of C3—4). *See* Appendix.

The external carotid lies on a line from the bifurcation, to a point immediately in front of the tragus behind the neck of the mandible, and passing behind the angle of the mandible. Here it divides into the *maxillary* and *superficial temporal arteries*. It gives off the *superior thyroid artery* (to thyroid gland) at the upper border of the thyroid cartilage, the *lingual artery* supplying the tongue at the level of the thyroid, and the *facial artery* immediately above the lingual, supplying the cheeks and lips. This crosses the mandible superficially 3 cm (1³⁄₁₆ in) anteriorly to the angle of the mandible. The *occipital artery*, arising immediately above the hyoid, runs backwards to supply the scalp.

The *superficial temporal artery* can be felt close to the pre-auricular point and divides 5 cm (2 in) above this point into anterior and posterior branches supplying the scalp.

The *maxillary artery* runs forwards behind the neck of the mandible to supply the maxilla and facial muscles.

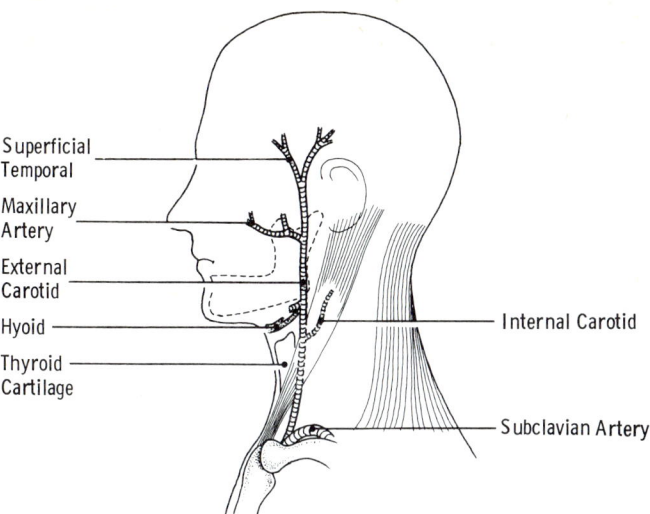

Superficial Temporal

Maxillary Artery

External Carotid

Hyoid

Thyroid Cartilage

Internal Carotid

Subclavian Artery

Fig. 20. Carotid arteries.

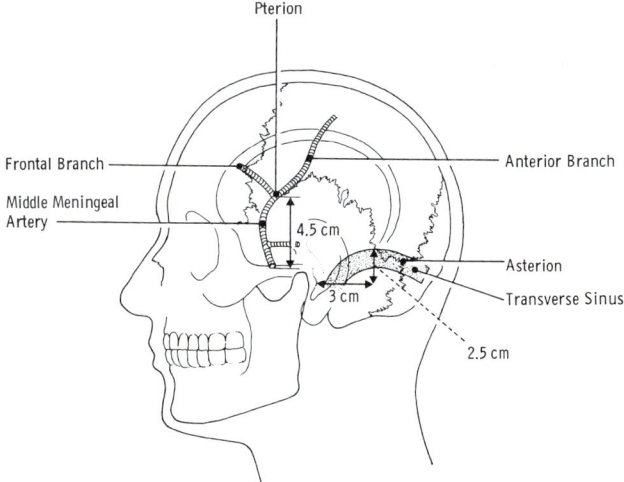

Pterion

Frontal Branch

Middle Meningeal Artery

Anterior Branch

4.5 cm

Asterion

Transverse Sinus

3 cm

2.5 cm

Fig. 21. Vessels of skull. (*After A.K.M.*)

The *middle meningeal artery* is a branch of the maxillary artery. It passes through the foramen spinosum into the skull, opposite the midpoint of the zygomatic arch, where it divides into anterior and posterior divisions. The anterior division runs vertically for 4·5 cm (1¾ in) to the pterion and then upwards and backwards towards a point on the vertex, midway between the glabella and the external occipital protuberance (inion). The posterior branch runs backwards towards the lambda (*Fig.* 21).

The *internal carotid artery* runs upwards to enter the skull through the carotid canal in the temporal bone. It lies on a line from the carotid bifurcation to the posterior border of the mandibular condyle. It supplies the anterior two-thirds of the brain, joining up with the opposite internal carotid and the vertebral arteries via the *Circle of Willis* and the *basilar artery* at the base of the brain. The *vertebral artery* originates from the subclavian artery and runs upwards in the neck postero-laterally through the foramina in the transverse processes of the cervical vertebrae, from C6 to C1. It enters the foramen of C6 at the level of the cricoid cartilage. It is accompanied by the vertebral vein.

VENOUS SINUSES OF THE SKULL AND VEINS OF NECK AND MEDIASTINUM

The *superior sagittal sinus* follows the sagittal suture of the skull, and is immediately deep to that suture. It commences at the glabella and continues backwards to the level of the inion (external occipital protuberance) where it drains into the right or left transverse sinus and communicates with the opposite transverse sinus and the straight sinus (running backwards in the midline, across the tentorium cerebelli). This point is called the *torcular Herophili,* or confluence of the sinuses.

The *transverse sinus* commences at the inion and runs laterally along the base of the cerebral hemisphere across the asterion to a point opposite the base of the mastoid process (*Fig.* 21). Here it turns downwards close to the posterior border of the process, to a point 1·2 cm (½ in) from its tip, where it leaves the skull through the jugular foramen, and becomes the *internal jugular vein*. This vein may be represented by a line from the lobule of the ear, to the sternal end of the clavicle, where it joins the subclavian vein to form the brachiocephalic vein (*Fig.* 26).

The *external jugular vein* drains venous blood from the outside of the scalp and face, commencing immediately below the angle of the mandible, running down the neck on a line from the angle of the mandible to the middle of the clavicle. It may be seen crossing the sternomastoid muscle and it drains into the subclavian vein.

The *brachiocephalic veins* (right and left) formed by the junction of the internal jugular and subclavian veins, commence behind the right and left sternoclavicular joints and run downwards and medially, to meet behind the sternal end of the first right intercostal space (*Fig.* 26). Here they form:

The *superior vena cava,* which runs vertically downwards alongside the sternal border, behind the second costal cartilage and second interspace, to enter the right atrium behind the third right costal cartilage. It is 2 cm (¾ in) wide.

The *inferior vena cava* passes through the diaphragm to enter the thorax at the level of the 8th and 9th thoracic vertebrae, immediately to the right of the mid-plane opposite the sternal end of the right 6th costal cartilage. It terminates in the heart at the level of the xiphisternal joint (T9) 2·5 cm (1 in) to the right of the midline.

Chapter 10

The thorax

The upper margin of the thorax is formed by the plane of the upper borders of the first pair of ribs and the first thoracic vertebra, passing through the disc space at C7–T1. This plane was formerly designated the *'thoracic inlet'*, but is now named the *superior thoracic aperture.*

The *inferior thoracic aperture* (thoracic outlet) is situated at the level of the T12–L1 disc space posteriorly, and the attachment of the diaphragm to the ribs and costal cartilages laterally, extending round to the tip of the xiphisternum anteriorly (*see* Appendix).

The *thorax* contains the heart and great vessels, the trachea and bronchi, the lungs and the oesophagus.

The *principal muscles of the chest wall* include:

The *pectoralis* which covers the anterior and lateral chest walls. It originates by digitations attached to the ribs and costal cartilages, anteriorly. These can be seen in a thin subject (*Plate* 3). The muscle consists of a thin sheet of muscle fibres extending laterally and upwards to be inserted into the anterior surface of the upper third of the humerus. Its lower border forms the anterior axillary fold. Posteriorly, the chest wall is covered by the trapezius and latissimus dorsi muscles. The latter originates from the spinous process of the lower thoracic vertebrae and the posterior surfaces of the ribs. It also extends down as far as the iliac crest. It extends upwards and laterally, to be inserted into the posterior surface of the humerus in the upper third and with teres major, forms the posterior fold of the axilla (*Plate* 10).

The *serratus anterior* muscle covers the upper and lateral parts of the thoracic wall. It arises from the outer surfaces and upper borders of the upper eight or nine ribs, and the aponeuroses over their intercostal muscles. It is inserted into the vertebral border and inferior angle of the scapula. It forms the medial wall of the axilla (*Plate* 10).

REFERENCE LINES OF THE THORAX

The *midclavicular* line is self explanatory, and is a vertical line drawn through the midpoint of the clavicle, parallel to the midplane. In most subjects it is about 9 cm ($3\frac{1}{2}$ in) from the midplane.

The *anterior and posterior axillary* lines are vertical lines corresponding with the anterior and posterior folds of the axilla. The *midaxillary* line lies halfway between them.

The *mediastinum* is the septum situated in the median plane, which divides the thorax into right and left halves. It consists of:

Superior mediastinum, extending from the superior thoracic aperture (thoracic inlet) on the plane of the first ribs, to a plane at the level of the lower margin of the manubrium sterni to the fourth thoracic vertebra, above the heart (*see* Appendix).

Inferior mediastinum, below this plane, to the diaphragm, divided into three parts:

1. *Anterior mediastinum* – in front of the heart.
2. *Middle mediastinum* – containing the heart and great vessels.
3. *Posterior mediastinum* – behind the heart.

The mediastinum separates the right and left lungs and pleura, and in addition to the heart, pericardium and great vessels, it contains:

1. The trachea and right and left main bronchi.
2. The oesophagus.
3. The thymus gland.
4. The phrenic and vagus nerves.
5. Lymphatic glands, lymphatic channels and thoracic duct.

SURFACE MARKINGS OF THE MEDIASTINUM

Superior Mediastinum: The median plane from the superior

margin of the sternum to the lower margin of the manubrium sterni (opposite T4) or sternal angle.

Anterior and Posterior Mediastinum: Also lie in the median plane, from the sternal angle to the level of the diaphragm at the xiphisternal joint (T9–10) (*see* Appendix).

Middle Mediastinum: Corresponds to the outline of the heart and pericardium (*see* below).

SURFACE MARKINGS OF THE MAJOR INTRATHORACIC ORGANS

The Oesophagus: The oesophagus commences at the lower border of the cricoid cartilage in the neck opposite C6 and is represented by two vertical lines 2·5 cm (1 in) apart. The upper part inclines to the left in the neck and enters the thorax opposite the left side of the body of T1 reaching the midline at the sternal angle (2nd costal cartilages) and then deviates to the left to the 7th costal cartilage 2·5 cm (1 in) to the left of the midplane, where it enters the stomach, at the cardiac orifice (*Fig.* 22).

The Trachea: The trachea commences at lower border of cricoid (opposite C6) and ends at level of sternal angle (T5) dividing into the right and left bronchi. It lies behind the midline of the sternum down to the bifurcation, where it is slightly (1 cm ($\frac{7}{16}$ in)) to the right of the midline (*Fig.* 23 and Appendix).

The Pericardium and Heart: These are situated behind the body of the sternum and the cartilages of the 2nd–6th ribs, and are outlined as follows:

Apex of heart – in 5th intercostal space 9 cm ($3\frac{1}{2}$ in) to the left of midline.

Right border – a line from upper border of 2nd right costal cartilage 3·7 cm ($1\frac{3}{4}$ in) from midline to the 6th costal cartilage, convex to the right.

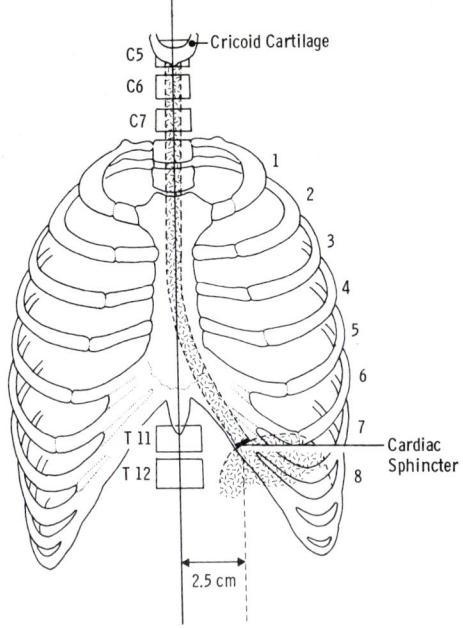

Fig. 22. Oesophagus.

Lower border — a line from right border to apex.

Left border — from apex up to lower border of 2nd left costal cartilage 3·7 cm (1½ in) from midline.

Base — complete upper border.

Aortic valve — behind middle of left half of sternum at level of 3rd intercostal space.

Mitral valve — behind sternal end of left 3rd intercostal space (or 4th costal cartilage) (*Fig.* 24).

Aorta

1. Ascending: commences at aortic valve at level of lower border of 3rd left costal cartilage behind left half of sternum.

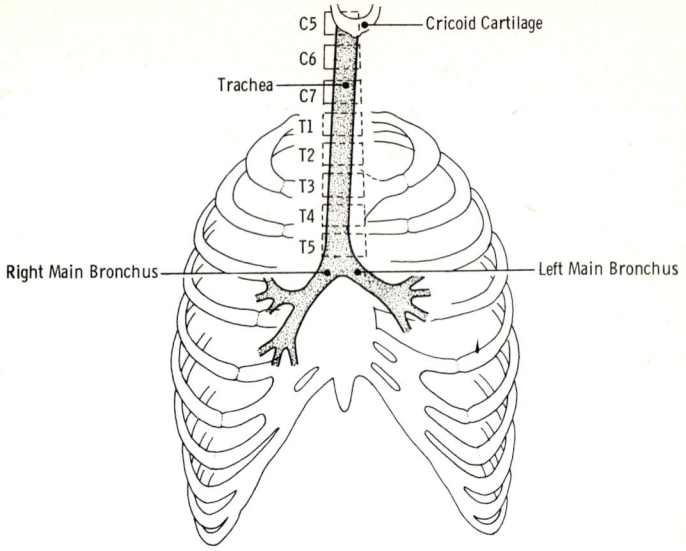

Fig. 23. Trachea and bronchi.

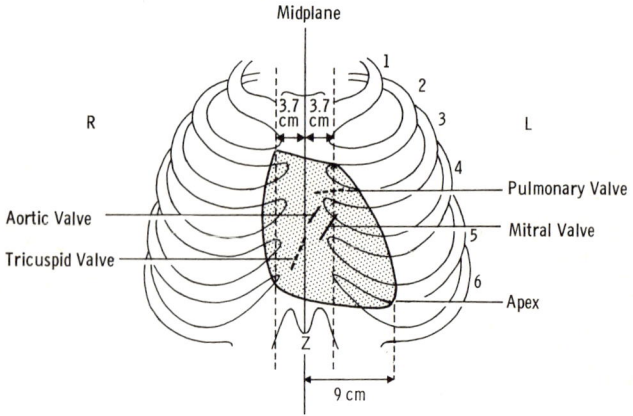

Fig. 24. Heart.

Passes upwards and to the right to level of upper border of 2nd right costal cartilage.

2. Arch: behind manubrium sterni at level of upper border of 2nd costal cartilages, running from right to left.

3. Descending thoracic aorta: from 2nd left costal cartilage downwards close to sternum, along a line reaching the midline at a point 8 cm (3 in) below the xiphisternal joint.

4. Abdominal aorta: continues from this point on a line downwards to a point slightly to the left of the midline, just above and to the left of the umbilicus (*Figs.* 25 and 27).

Branches of the Aorta: The main branches of the thoracic aorta are as follows:

1. Right and Left Coronary Arteries.
These arise from the ascending aorta, at its root, close to the aortic valve.

The right coronary artery runs vertically downwards and slightly to the right, from the aortic valve (3rd intercostal space) close to the midplane, and crossing it at the lower border of the heart, behind the xiphisternal joint. It supplies the right atrium and right ventricle.

The left coronary artery passes to the left behind the pulmonary artery to reach the left heart border, and then descends close to that border, to the heart apex. It supplies the left atrium, left ventricle and right ventricle.

2. Brachiocephalic (or Innominate) Artery.
Arises from the arch of the aorta, in the midline, behind the sternal angle (2nd costal cartilage level). It runs upwards and to the right, to a point behind the right sternoclavicular joint, where it divides into the right subclavian and right common carotid arteries. It is 4—5 cm ($1\frac{1}{2}$ —2 in) long (*Fig.* 25).

3. The Left Common Carotid, and
4. Left Subclavian Arteries.
These arise from the aortic arch close to the left border of the sternum, at the level of the sternal angle (2nd left costal cartilage region).

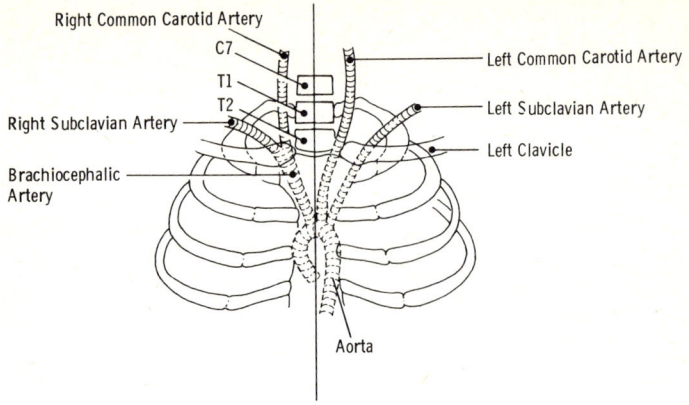

Fig. 25. Arteries of thoracic inlet.

The subclavian artery can be represented by a line convex upwards, from the sternoclavicular joint to the midpoint of the clavicle, rising to 2 cm (¾ in) above it (*Fig.* 25).

5. Intercostal Arteries

Intercostal Arteries (9 pairs) are given off from the descending thoracic aorta at each intercostal space, and run around the chest wall in the intercostal spaces, along the lower borders of the lower nine ribs.

The *main pulmonary artery* can be represented by two parallel lines 2·5 cm (1 in) apart, drawn from the pulmonary valve (behind the medial end of the 3rd left intercostal space) upwards and to the left, to the 2nd left costal cartilage. Here it divides into the right and left pulmonary arteries, running laterally right and left to the lung roots.

The *right pulmonary artery* crosses the midline in front of the 6th thoracic vertebra, and in front of the right main bronchus, behind the ascending aorta, at the 4th rib level.

The *pulmonary veins* (two on each side) accompany the pulmonary arteries on either side, from the lung roots to the left atrium.

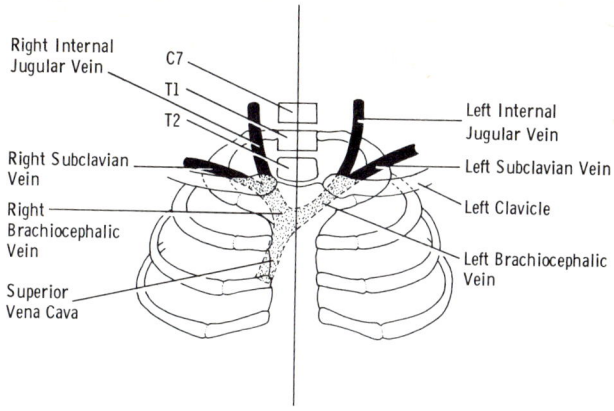

Fig. 26. Veins of thoracic inlet.

Ultrasound scanning of the heart is performed by means of T–P ('time–position') scan with a cardiac probe.

To obtain echoes from the mitral valve, the probe is directed slightly medially and upwards towards the right shoulder, in the 3rd left interspace. The probe is then moved slowly laterally. If no echoes are picked up, the 4th and 5th interspaces may be tried. Rotating the patient towards the left may help.

For the aortic valve scan, after obtaining the mitral scan, angle the probe more medially and towards the head. (*See Ultrasonics in Clinical Diagnosis* Ed. P. N. T. Wells.)

Lungs and Pleura
1. Lungs

Apices: Anteriorly – on a convex line above the medial third of the clavicle, extending 2·5 cm (1 in) upwards into the neck on quiet respiration.

Posteriorly – at the level of T1, 5 cm (2 in) from the midline (*Fig.* 28).

Posterior borders – on a line 2 cm ($\frac{3}{4}$ in) from the mid-

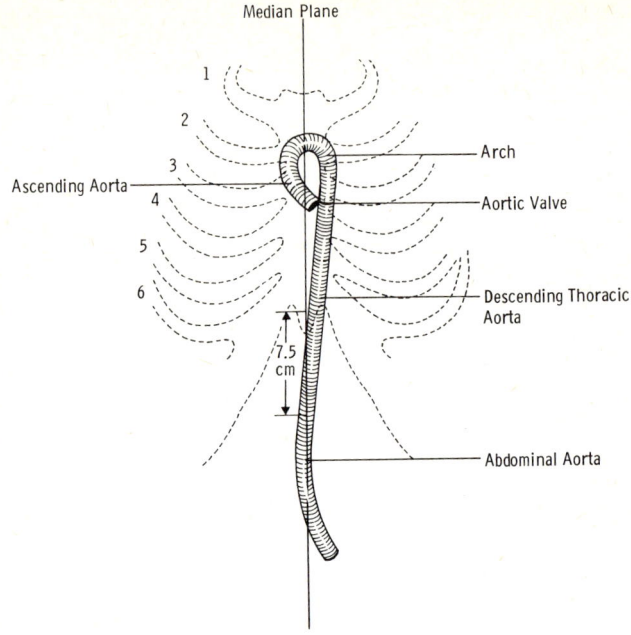

Fig. 27. Thoracic aorta.

line from the level of the spinous processes of T2 to T10—11 vertically.

Anterior borders — on a line running vertically downwards from the sternoclavicular joints, close together behind the manubrium sterni to the level of the 4th costal cartilages.

On the right side — joins inferior border behind the 6th right chrondrosternal joint.

On the left side — the anterior border of the left lung shows a notch (cardiac notch) represented by a concave line from the 4th left chrondrosternal joint to a point on the 6th costal cartilage 2·5 cm (1 in) from the edge of the sternum.

Inferior borders — move up and down on respiration 5—7½ cm (2—3 in). From anterior end of 6th costal cartilages

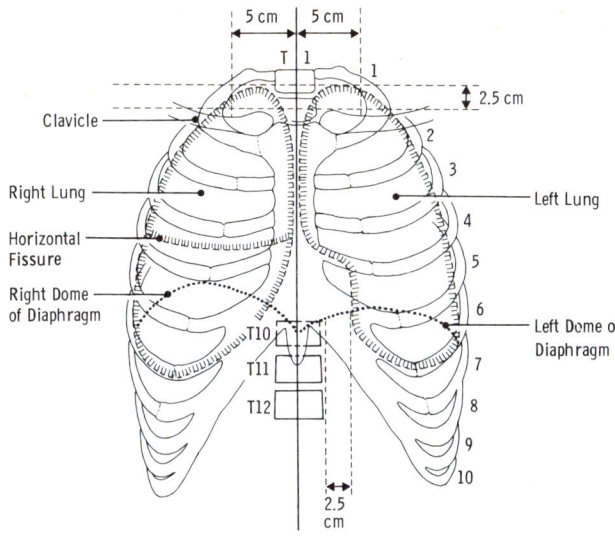

Fig. 28. Lungs and pleura: anterior view.

to the lowest points of the 6th costal cartilages, thence horizontally around sides of the thorax to the interval between spinous processes of T10–11.

2. Pleura

Similar to the lungs but just medial to the medial borders of the lungs except at the cardiac notch.

The mediastinal line of reflection of the left pleura is represented by a line running downwards, immediately to the left of the sternal border to the 7th left costal cartilage.

The diaphragmatic lines of reflection are represented by lines from the junction of the sternal and diaphragmatic lines to a point 5 cm (2 in) above the lowest point of the 10th costal cartilages, backwards horizontally through the inter-section of the 12th ribs with the lateral margin of the

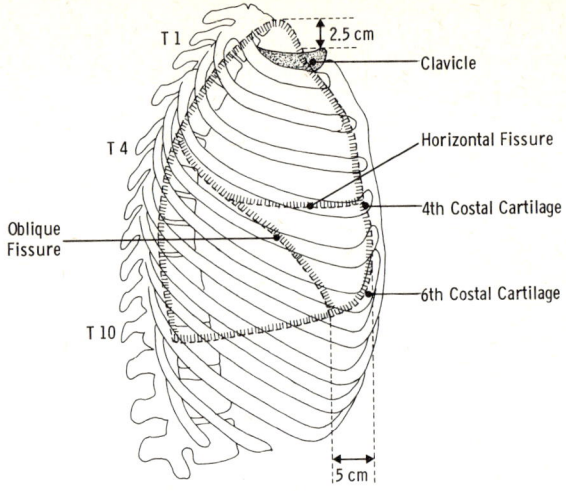

Fig. 29. Lungs and pleura: right lateral view. (*After A.K.M.*)

sacrospinalis muscles then medially they extend below the 12th ribs to the spinous process of L1.

The lungs have segments, each with a bronchus to it, and fissures separate the segments.

Right lung – three lobes, separated by oblique and horizontal fissures.

Left lung – two lobes. The lingula segment belongs to the left upper lobe (*Fig.* 28).

The *oblique fissure* lies on a line commencing posteriorly at the level of the spinous process of T3, passing obliquely forwards around the side of the chest wall following the 6th rib, and reaching the inferior border of the lung at the 6th costal cartilage 5 cm (2 in) from the margin of the sternum.

The *horizontal fissure* of the right lung corresponds with a horizontal line at the level of the 4th right costal cartilage. This line meets the oblique fissure in the posterior axillary line (*Fig.* 29).

Chapter 11

The abdomen

The abdomen has only a few bony landmarks, such as the costal margins, the iliac crests and spines, and the symphysis pubis, to which the internal organs can be related. It is therefore divided into regions, by using several vertical and horizontal planes as follows:

1. *Transpyloric plane:* A horizontal plane situated midway between the jugular notch (upper margin of sternum) and the symphysis pubis.

2. *Subcostal plane:* A horizontal plane situated at the lowest points of the costal margins.

3. *Transtubercular plane:* A horizontal plane at the level of the tubercles on the iliac crests at the level of the 5th lumbar spinous process.

4. *Lateral planes:* Vertical planes on either side of the median plane, passing through the midpoints of the inguinal ligaments (which extend from the anterior superior iliac spines to the symphysis pubis). These divide the abdomen into regions as shown in *Fig.* 30.

Other planes which are frequently used in abdominal surface markings are the *supracristal plane,* at the level of the highest point of the iliac crests (usually opposite the 4th lumbar spine) and the *interspinous plane,* passing through the anterior superior iliac spines (*see* Appendix).

MUSCLES OF THE ABDOMINAL WALL (*Plate* 4)

The *linea alba* is a fibrous band forming a shallow depression in the midline of the abdomen, extending from the xiphisternum to the symphysis pubis.

On either side of it, forming visible ridges are the two *rectus*

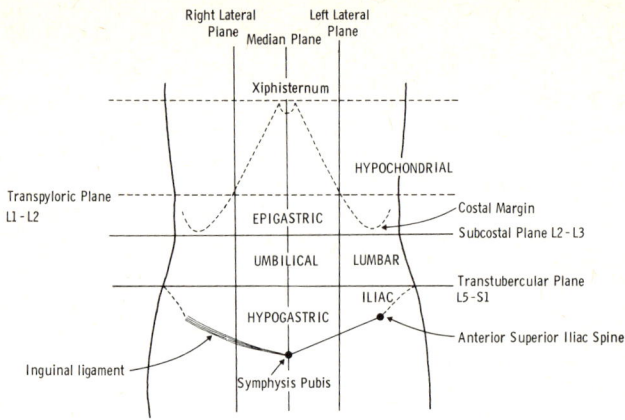

Fig. 30. Regions and planes of the abdomen.

abdominis muscles originating from the superior margins of the pubic bones medially, and inserted into the xiphisternum and the cartilages of the 5th, 6th and 7th ribs. Each muscle is enclosed in a fibrous sheath which has a curved groove along its lateral margin, called the *linea semilunaris*. This groove meets the costal margin, above, at the tip of the 9th costal cartilage, and the pubic crest, below, at the *pubic tubercle* (*Fig.* 31 and *Plate* 4).

The linea semilunaris approximates with the *lateral plane* of the abdomen (*see* planes of the abdomen).

The lower margin of the rectus sheath forms a curved line inferiorly and posteriorly, called the *linea semicircularis*, situated on a line midway between the umbilicus and the symphysis pubis (*Plate* 4).

The anterior abdominal wall also contains:

1. The *external oblique* muscles, originating from the lower ribs, running downwards and forwards to be inserted into the iliac crests and the linea alba (*Fig.* 31).

2. The *internal oblique* muscles, deep to the external

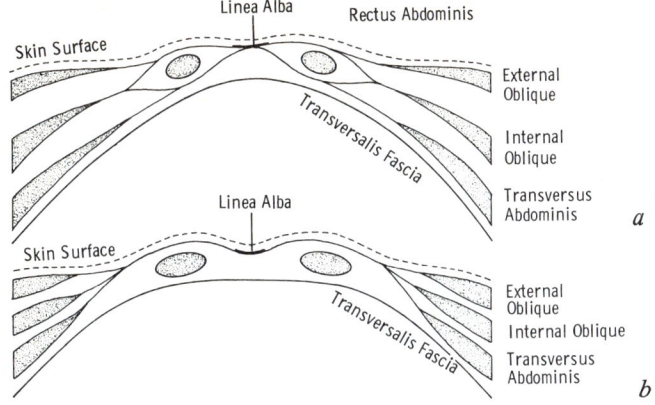

Fig. 31. Transverse sections of abdominal wall (*a*) through
the rectus sheath; (*b*) below the linea semicircularis.

obliques, which originate from the iliac crests and run upwards
and inwards, to be inserted into the lower ribs and linea alba.

3. The *transversus abdominis* muscles, which lie deepest,
originating from the iliac crests, the transverse processes of the
lumbar vertebrae and the fibrous sheaths around the quadratus
lumborum muscles (*Fig.* 32). They are inserted into the linea
alba centrally. Their fibres run transversely across the abdomen.

Each of these muscles forms an *aponeurosis* (a flat white
fibrous tendon-like sheet) over the anterior abdominal wall.
They are arranged in layers as shown in *Fig.* 31 (*a*) above, and
lower down below the linea semicircularis, as shown in *Fig.*
31 (*b*).

In the *posterior wall* of the abdomen on either side of the
lumbar spine, are the following muscles:

1. *Sacrospinalis,* on either side of the *median spinal furrow,*
which is situated over the lumbar spinous processes. The
sacrospinalis muscles form distinct ridges running vertically up

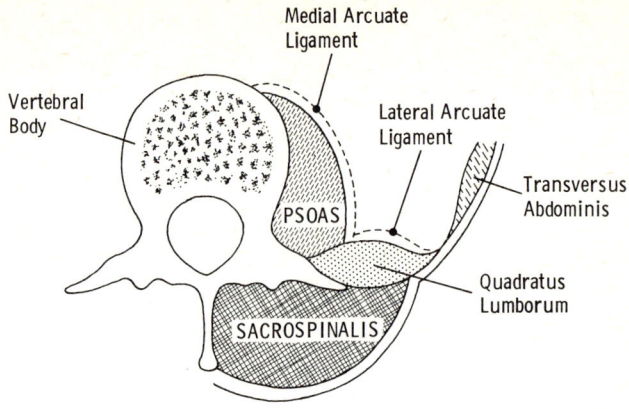

Fig. 32. Transverse section of lumbar **muscles.**

and back from the iliac crests and sacrum, into the thoracic region (*Plate* 7).

They are bounded laterally by palpable grooves along the outer borders of the sacrospinalis muscles. These extend upwards from a point lateral to the posterior superior iliac spines, to the 12th ribs.

2. *Quadratus lumborum,* situated lateral to the sacrospinalis, originating from the iliac crest posteriorly, and inserted into the lower ribs.

3. *Psoas,* alongside the bodies of the lumbar vertebrae anteriorly to their transverse processes, from which it originates. These muscles run downwards (on either side) through the pelvis, merging with the *iliacus* muscles. They are inserted via a tendon passing deep to the inguinal ligament, to the lesser trochanter of the femur. Crossing the psoas muscle is the *medial arcuate ligament* attached to the sides of the bodies of the 1st and 2nd lumbar vertebrae and the crura of the diaphragm medially, and laterally to the transverse process of the 1st lumbar vertebra.

The quadratus lumborum passes similarly beneath the

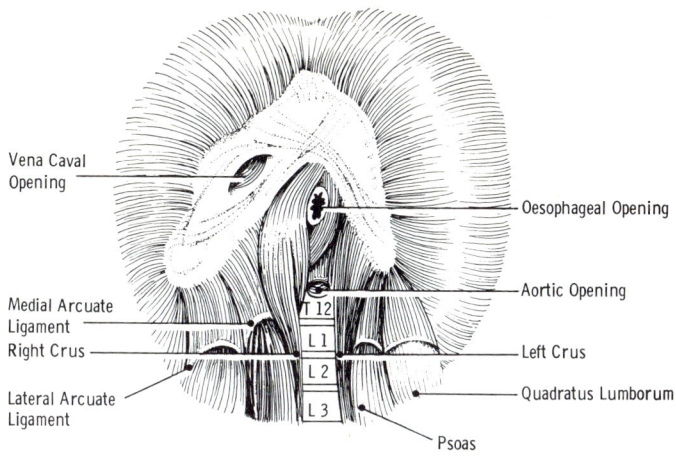

Fig. 33. Diaphragm.

lateral arcuate ligament attached medially to the transverse process of L1 and laterally to the lower margin of the 12th rib (*Fig. 32*).

The *diaphragm* consists of a dome-shaped fibromuscular structure, separating the abdomen from the thorax (*Fig. 33*).

Radiating muscle fibres extend from the thoracic wall to a central tendon, or aponeurosis, shaped like a clover leaf, into which it is inserted.

It originates (1) anteriorly from the posterior surface of the xiphisternum; (2) laterally from the inner surfaces of the lower six ribs and costal cartilages; (3) posteriorly (*a*) by 2 crura from the anterior surfaces of 1st, 2nd and 3rd lumbar vertebrae, on the right side, and from the 1st and 2nd lumbar vertebrae, on the left side; (*b*) from the medial and lateral arcuate ligaments bridging over the psoas and quadratus lumborum muscles.

The crura surround three openings, situated posteriorly, these are:

1. *Aortic* opening, which is the most posterior and

lowest, at the level of the 12th thoracic or 1st lumbar vertebrae.

2. *Oesophageal* opening, above, and in front of, and to the left of the aortic opening, at the level of T10.

3. *Vena caval* opening, which is the highest opening in front of the oesophageal opening, and at the level of 8th and 9th thoracic vertebrae. (*See* Appendix and *Fig.* 33.)

SURFACE MARKINGS OF THE MAJOR ABDOMINAL ORGANS

STOMACH

The stomach lies in the left upper quadrant of abdominal cavity.

Supine: Cardiac orifice lies behind 7th left costal cartilage 2·5 cm (1 in) to the left of median plane (opposite T11–12). *Pylorus* lies on transpyloric plane 1·2 cm ($\frac{1}{2}$ in) to right of median plane. *Lesser curve* lies on a J-shaped line from the cardiac orifice to the pylorus. *Fundus* corresponds with a line convex upwards from cardiac orifice to the left, reaching its summit in the left 5th intercostal space. *Greater curve* – a curved line convex to the left downwards from the fundus to the pylorus, cutting the left costal margin between the tips of the 9th and 10th costal cartilages, extending down to the subcostal plane (*Fig.* 34*a*).

Erect: In the erect position, the cardiac orifice descends from the level of the upper border of T12 to the upper border of L1 (7th costal cartilage to 8th costal cartilage). The pylorus and 1st stage of duodenum drop from the level of the spinous process of L1 to the level of the upper border of L4 (supra-cristal plane). The fundus extends up to the level of the 6th left interspace (*Fig.* 34*b*).

DUODENUM

The duodenum lies entirely above the umbilicus. About 2·5 cm (1 in) wide.

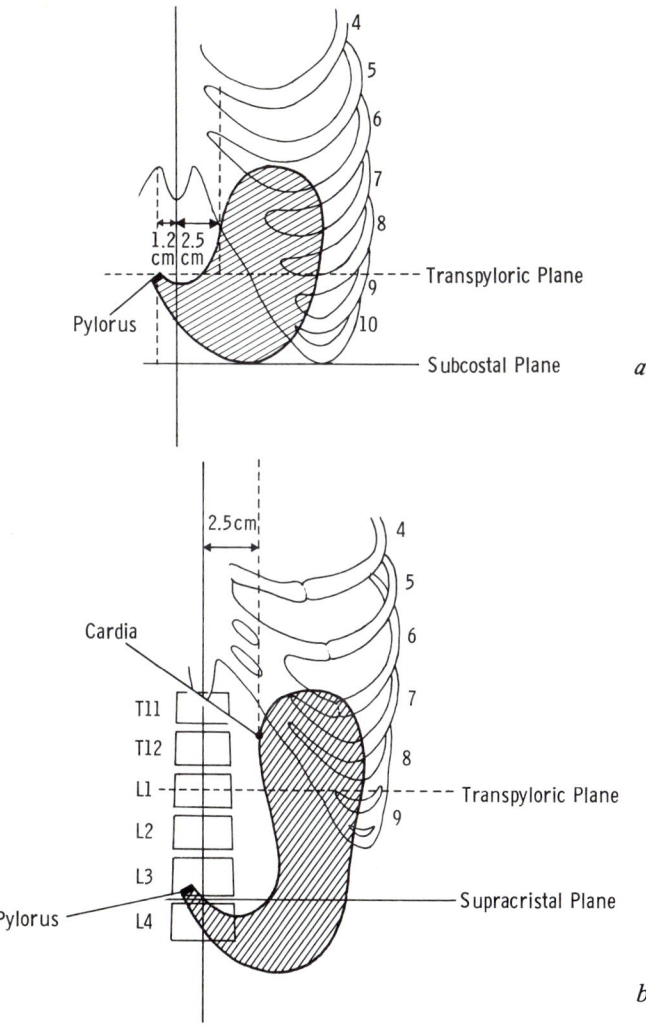

Fig. 34. Stomach: (*a*) Supine; (*b*) Erect.

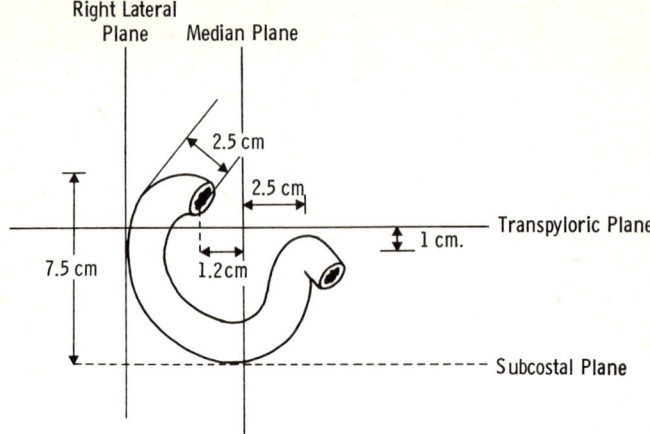

Fig. 35. Duodenum.

First Stage: Upwards to the right 2·5 cm (1 in) from the pylorus.

Second Stage: Descends downwards for 7·5 cm (3 in) lying medial to the right lateral plane.

Third Stage: Horizontal from lower end of descending part, transversely to the left, above the umbilicus and after crossing the median plane it turns upwards into *fourth stage* (ascending stage), which ends at the duodenojejunal junction situated 2·5 cm (1 in) to left of median plane and 1 cm (½ in) below transpyloric plane (*Fig.* 35).

PANCREAS

The pancreas stretches obliquely across posterior abdominal wall, lying more to left (than right) of median plane, over L1 and 2.

Head lies within the loop of the duodenum. Its neck extends upwards and to the left behind the pylorus.

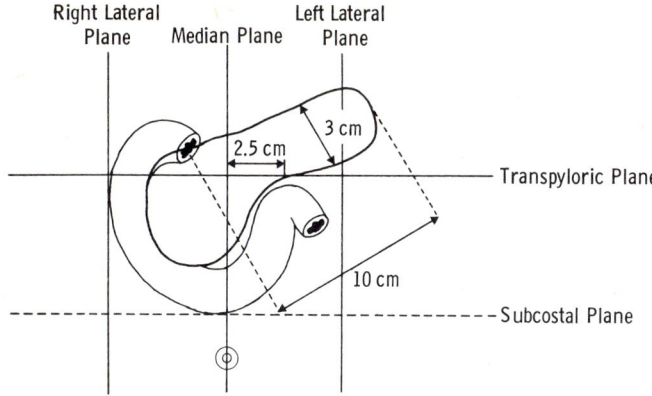

Right Lateral
Plane   Median Plane
Left Lateral
Plane

3 cm

2.5 cm

Transpyloric Plane

10 cm

Subcostal Plane

Fig. 36. Pancreas.

Body represented by two parallel lines 3 cm (1¼ in) apart drawn upwards and to the left for 10–12 cm (4–5 in) from the neck (*Fig.* 36).

LIVER

The liver occupies right upper quadrant of abdomen, roughly triangular. Upper border corresponds to a line drawn through the xiphisternal joint and ascending to a point 1 cm (½ in) below the right nipple (5th intercostal space) and ascending less sharply to the left to a point 2·5 cm (1 in) below, and medial to the left nipple (8 cm (3¼ in) from the midline).

The right border corresponds to a curved line convex to the right drawn from right end of upper border to a point 1 cm (½ in) below right costal margin at tip of right 10th costal cartilage, and at the level of the 6th right rib in the midaxillary line. The lower border joins the remaining two ends and crosses the median plane at the transpyloric plane level (*Fig.* 37).

SPLEEN

The spleen lies in the left hypochondrium posteriorly, close to the 9th, 10th and 11th ribs. The medial end is 5 cm

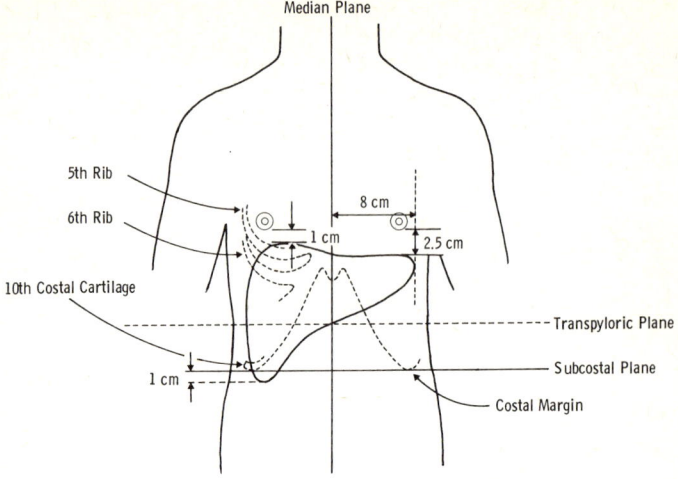

Fig. 37. Liver.

(2 in) from the midline and its long axis lies along the
10th rib, extending around to the midaxillary line. It may
be scanned ultrasonically through the 10th interspace
(*Fig.* 38).

GALLBLADDER

Fundus at the angle between right costal margin and the lateral
border of right rectus muscle (linea semilunaris).

The *common bile duct* commences 2·5 cm (1 in) to the
right of the midline in the 6th intercostal space and runs
downwards and inwards to the costal margin. It then runs
parallel to the midline for 4 cm (1½ in) and then downwards
and laterally for 2 cm (¾ in) where it curves around the second
stage of duodenum. It is approximately 7·5 cm (3 in) long, and
its lower end lies 1·75 cm (⅝ in) from the midplane on the
subcostal plane. The portal vein and hepatic artery accompany
it (*Figs.* 39 and 40).

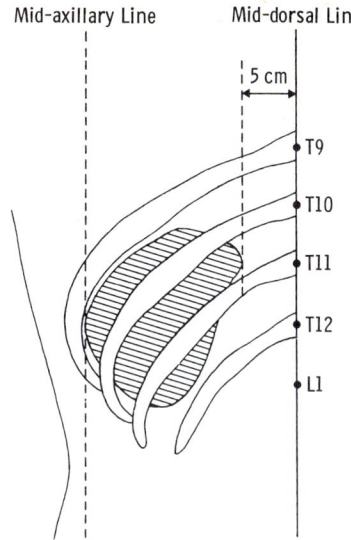

Fig. 38. Spleen.

SMALL INTESTINE

The small intestine is continuous with the duodenum and consists of the jejunum and ileum, opening into the large intestine at the ileocaecal valve. They are situated in the umbilical and hypogastric regions, bounded by the ascending colon, stomach and descending colon. It ends at the *ileocaecal valve* which is located at the point where the right lateral and transtubercular planes intersect.

COLON

Caecum and Appendix are situated in triangular area between right lateral and transtubercular planes, and inguinal ligament (right iliac region) (*Fig.* 41).

Ascending Colon – 5 cm (2 in) wide, ascends from transtubercular plane, immediately to right of right lateral plane to

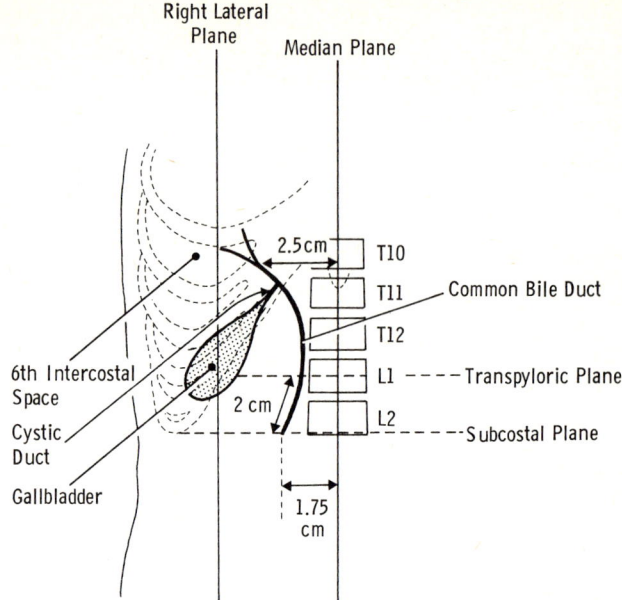

Fig. 39. Gallbladder and bile ducts.

midway between subcostal and transpyloric planes (behind the right 9th costal cartilage).

Transverse Colon a band 5 cm (2 in) wide, from upper end of ascending colon, downwards and medially to the umbilicus, then laterally and upwards, crossing transpyloric plane to left of lateral plane (behind the left 8th costal cartilage).

Descending Colon – 2 cm ($\frac{3}{4}$ in) wide, commences above transpyloric plane and descends lateral to left lateral plane to inguinal ligament.

Pelvic Colon in hypogastrium behind the bladder.

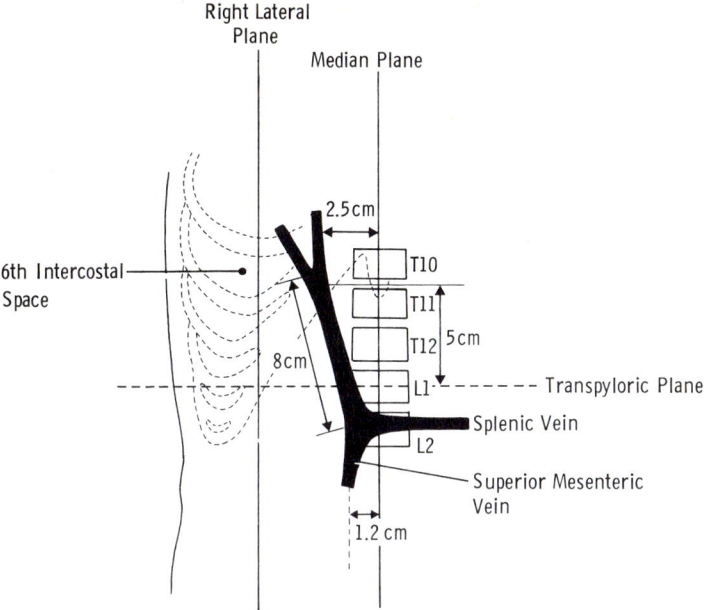

Fig. 40. Portal vein.

KIDNEYS

11 cm (4½ in) × 6·5 cm (2½ in) (posterior aspect (*Fig.* 42).
Upper and lateral parts situated under the costal margin
directed downwards and outwards, so that the upper poles are
2·5 cm (1 in) nearer the median plane, than the lower poles.

Hilum lies 5 cm (2 in) from midplane (right and left).

Right hilum just below, and left hilum just above transpyloric plane.

Inner borders are approximately 2·5 cm (1 in) and lateral
borders 9 cm (3½ in) from the midline respectively.

The upper poles of the kidneys are opposite the 11th
thoracic vertebral spine, and the lower poles opposite the spine
of the 3rd lumbar vertebra. The *suprarenal glands* overlie the
upper poles of the kidneys.

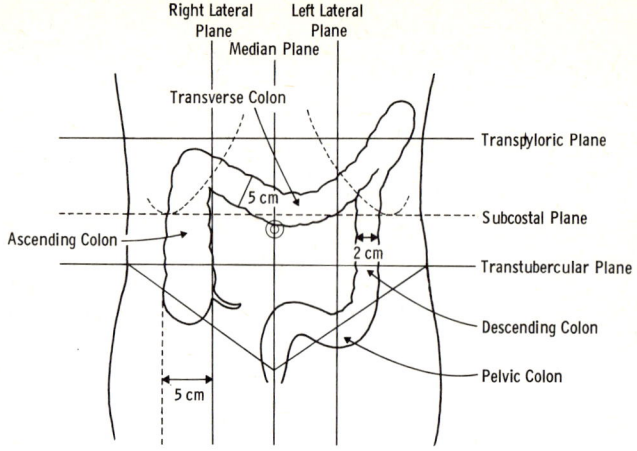

Fig. 41. Colon.

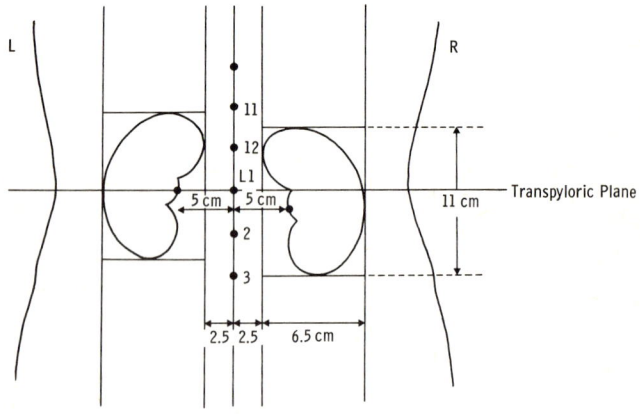

Fig. 42. Kidneys (posterior view).

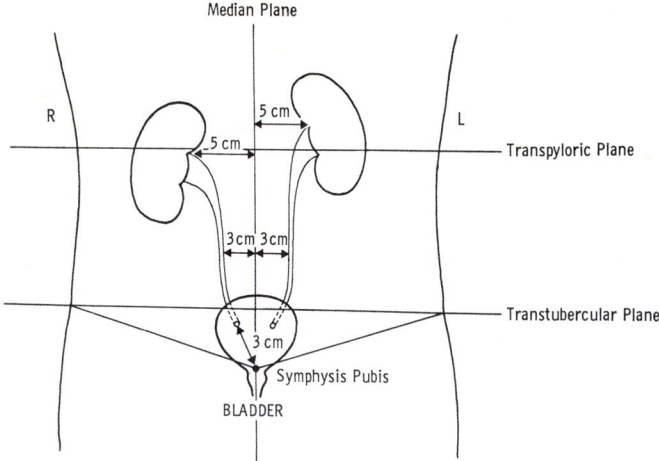

Fig. 43. Urinary tract.

URETERS

The ureters lie on either side of the midline, extending from the hila of the kidneys along a line to the point of entry into the pelvis. Here they are situated 3 cm (1¼ in) from the midline, on the transtubercular plane. They then turn medially, entering the bladder at a point 3 cm (1¼ in) lateral to the upper margin of the symphysis pubis (markings on the anterior abdominal wall).

BLADDER

The bladder is situated in the hypogastrium with lower border behind the symphysis pubis, and the fundus, extending up towards the umbilicus, when distended (*Fig.* 43).

UTERUS

The uterus lies behind the bladder and can be detected by ultrasound, through the filled bladder. Its cervix is immediately behind the upper border of the symphysis pubis, and the fundus on the interspinous plane.

During pregnancy it extends upwards into the hypogastric and umbilical regions, reaching the umbilicus at 24 weeks and the xiphisternal plane at 40 weeks.

OVARIES
The ovaries are situated on either side, at the level of the iliac spines (interspinous plane) immediately medial to the lateral vertical planes (*Fig.* 44).

VESSELS OF THE ABDOMEN
The *abdominal aorta* extends from the aortic orifice in the diaphragm, at the level of T12, to the bifurcation opposite L4, situated slightly to the left of the midline in the central abdomen, on the supracristal plane (*Fig.* 45).

MAIN BRANCHES OF THE ABDOMINAL AORTA
1. *Coeliac Artery* (1·25 cm, $\frac{1}{2}$ in long) arises from the front of the aorta immediately below the diaphragm at the level of the 12th thoracic vertebra, slightly to the left of the midplane (2·5 cm (1 in) above the transpyloric plane).

It divides into:

a. Gastric Artery – represented by a line from the coeliac artery, upwards and to the left, in the direction of the cardiac orifice (7th left costal cartilage).

b. Splenic Artery – on a line to the left, and slightly upwards, for 10 cm (4 in) from the coeliac artery.

c. Hepatic Artery – a line to the right and downwards from the coeliac artery for 2·5 cm (1 in) then vertically upwards for 2–3 cm ($\frac{3}{4}$–$1\frac{1}{4}$ in).

2. *Superior Mesenteric Artery* arises in the midline at the transpyloric plane 1 cm ($\frac{1}{2}$ in) below the coeliac artery (L1–2). Its course corresponds to the root of the mesentery: a line drawn downwards and to the right from this point to the intersection of the transtubercular and right lateral planes.

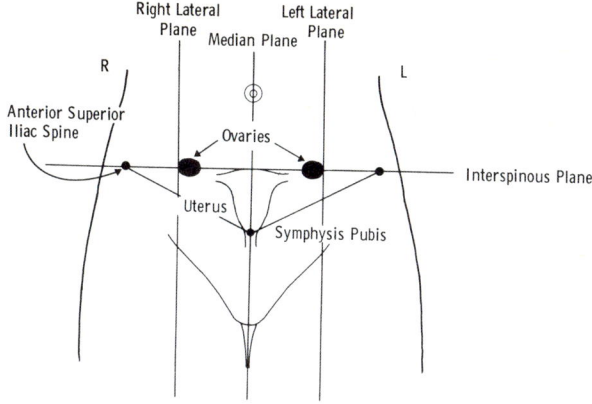

Fig. 44. Uterus and ovaries.

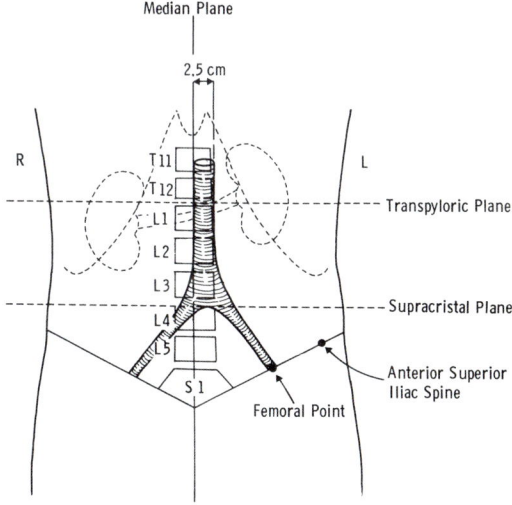

Fig. 45. Abdominal aorta.

3. The *Renal Arteries* arise from the aorta laterally 1·5 cm ($\frac{1}{2}$ in) below the transpyloric plane in front of L2. They are about 4 cm ($1\frac{1}{2}$ in) long extending horizontally on either side of the aorta to the kidneys.

4. The *Inferior Mesenteric Artery* arises about 3 cm ($1\frac{1}{4}$ in) above the supracristal plane (L2—3) and runs downwards and to the left for 6·5 cm ($2\frac{1}{2}$ in).

The *common iliac arteries* commence at the bifurcation of the aorta (*see above*) and lie on a line running downwards and outwards towards the femoral points (on either side); midway between the anterior superior iliac spines and the symphysis pubis (*Fig.* 45).

The common iliac arteries divide into *external and internal iliac arteries* at a point one-third of the way down this line, continuing as the external iliac arteries, to the level of the inguinal ligaments.

The *inferior vena cava* lies parallel to the aorta, immediately to the right of the median plane, commencing 2·5 cm (1 in) below the supracristal plane and ending at a point 2·5 cm (1 in) to the right of the xiphisternal joint. It is formed by the junction of right and left common iliac veins.

The *portal vein* is formed by the junction of the splenic and superior mesenteric veins at the level of the 2nd lumbar vertebra (subcostal plane) about 1·2 cm ($\frac{1}{2}$ in) to the right of the midplane.

It runs to the right and upwards for 8 cm ($3\frac{1}{4}$ in) to enter the liver at the porta hepatis alongside the hepatic artery and common hepatic duct, 2·5 cm (1 in) to the right of the mid-plane, in the 6th right interspace, i.e. 5 cm (2 in) above the transpyloric plane (*Fig.* 40).

The *inferior mesenteric vein* drains into the splenic vein.

NOTES ON ULTRASOUND EXAMINATION OF THE ABDOMEN AND PELVIS

Ultrasound is widely used for examination of the pelvic

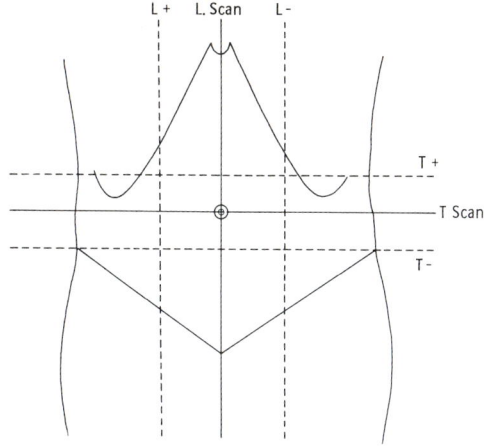

Fig. 46. Ultrasound scan diagram.

organs, particularly in pregnancy, and for examination of the liver, spleen, kidneys, gallbladder and aorta.

ULTRASOUND SCANS

Ultrasound scans of the abdomen and pelvis are carried out conventionally in the longitudinal and transverse directions, with the subject's head to the left in the longitudinal scan, and the subject supine (*Fig.* 46).

An 'L' scan is made in the longitudinal direction through the vertical median plane.

Scans to the right of the median plane are denoted by a '+' sign, and those to the left by a '−' sign, with the distance from the midline indicated in centimetres.

e.g. L + 1 indicates a longitudinal scan, 1 cm ($\frac{1}{2}$ in) to the right of the median plane, and L − 2 indicates a longitudinal scan 2 cm ($\frac{3}{4}$ in) to the left of the median plane.

Transverse scans are conventionally considered to be viewed from below: i.e. the right side of the scan is on the observer's left, and vice versa, with the subject supine.

A 'T' scan is made through the abdomen transversely, at the level of the umbilicus, with the distance above and below the umbilical level indicated by ' + ' and ' − ' signs.

e.g. T + 2 is a transverse scan through a horizontal plane 2 cm ($\frac{3}{4}$ in) above the umbilicus, and T − 3 a similar scan 3 cm ($1\frac{1}{4}$ in) below the umbilical level.

Renal scans are usually carried out with the subject prone, but are still considered to be viewed from below, so that the subject's right side is now on the observer's right. Longitudinal renal scans, although also performed with the subject prone, are labelled with the same convention as for the normal abdominal scan.

Scans of the liver are usually carried out along planes parallel to the costal margin, and designated by the distance from the costal margin in centimetres: 1 ($\frac{1}{2}$ in); 2 ($\frac{3}{4}$ in); and 3 cm ($1\frac{1}{4}$ in). The probe is directed upwards about 45° towards the thorax.

Chapter 12

The arm

1. MUSCLES OF THE SHOULDER AND UPPER ARM

The point of the shoulder is covered by the *deltoid* muscle originating from the spine of the scapula and the lateral third of the clavicle, and inserted into the lateral surface of the shaft of the humerus, half way down the shaft (deltoid impression).

It covers the head of the humerus, the tendons inserted into the tuberosities of the humerus (teres minor, supraspinatus, infraspinatus, and subscapularis) and also the tendon of the long head of the biceps muscle (*Fig.* 47 and *Plate* 5).

Calcification may occur in these tendons and in the sub-acromial bursa situated immediately below the acromion process.

The limits of the deltoid can be felt, when the arm is abducted to a horizontal position.

Anteriorly, the shoulder joint is crossed by the *pectoralis major* muscle, extending from the anterior chest wall to the anterior surface of the shaft of the humerus, below the greater tuberosity (bicipital groove). This muscle forms the anterior fold of the *axilla* (*Plates* 3 and 10). The posterior fold of the axilla is formed by the *latissimus dorsi* and *teres major* muscles, extending from the posterior chest wall and the inferior angle of scapula respectively to be inserted into the upper third of the humerus (medially to pectoralis major) (*Plate* 10) along the inner bicipital crest. The *serratus anterior* (magnus) muscle extends up from the chest wall to form the floor, or medial surface of the axilla. The shaft of the humerus is covered (*Plate* 5) by the *biceps* (*brachii*) and *brachialis* muscles anteriorly and laterally, and the *triceps* (*brachii*) medially. These originate from the scapula and shaft of

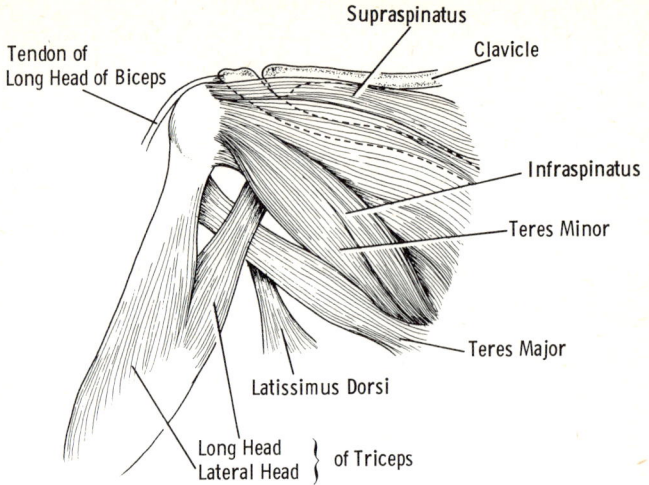

Fig. 47. Muscles around the shoulder.

humerus, and are inserted into the neck of the radius (biceps) and olecranon process of the ulna (triceps).

2. MUSCLES OF THE FOREARM AND HAND

The *extensor muscles* of the forearm, wrists and hand originate from the region of the lateral epicondyle of the humerus, and cover the posterior surface of the forearm (*Plate* 6).

The *flexor muscles* of the forearm, wrist and hand originate from the medial epicondyle, and cover the anterior surface of the forearm. These muscles are inserted, via tendons, into the carpal and metacarpal bones of the wrist and hand posteriorly for the extensors, and anteriorly for the flexors, respectively. Similarly the extensors and flexors of the fingers are inserted through tendons, into the phalanges (*Fig.* 48).

The *cubital fossa* is a hollow seen on the anterior aspect of the elbow, formed by the *brachialis, brachioradialis* and *extensor muscles* laterally, and the *pronator teres* and *flexor muscles* medially (*Fig.* 49).

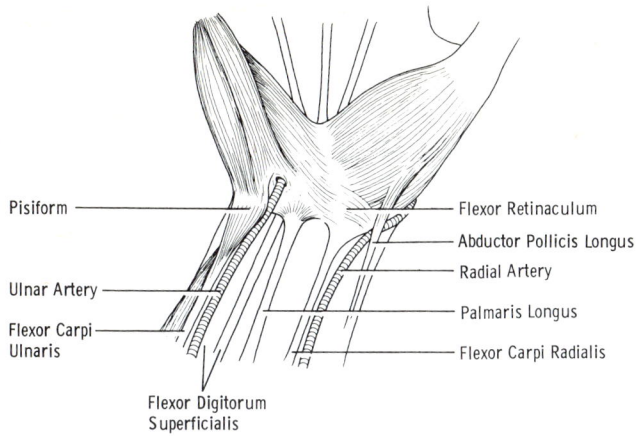

Fig. 48. Flexor tendons of wrist. (*After A.K.M.*)

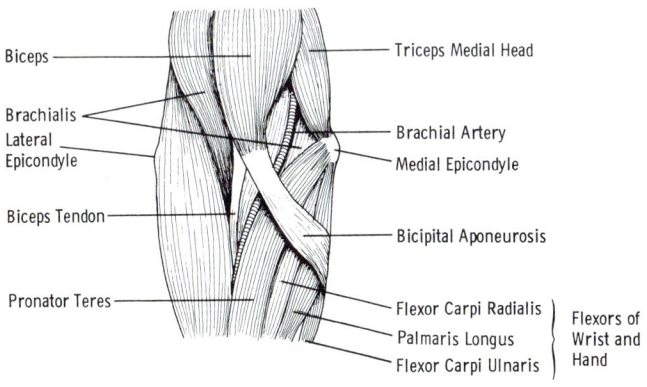

Fig. 49. Cubital fossa.

The *flexor tendons* may be seen and felt crossing the front of the wrist on flexing the wrist joint.

The most important of these are the *flexor carpi radialis* laterally, and the *palmaris longus,* which is situated in the midline of the wrist. The *flexor carpi ulnaris* is seen medially, on the ulnar side (*Fig.* 48) leading to the pisiform, into which it is inserted. These tendons are held in place by the *flexor retinaculum* a fibrous band attached to the scaphoid laterally, and the hamate and pisiform medially. The flexor tendons of wrist and fingers pass deep to it (i.e. flexor carpi ulnaris, flexor carpi radialis, flexor pollicis longus, flexor digitorum superficialis and flexor digitorum profundus). Palmaris longus tendon is partly inserted into it and also into the palmar fascia. The extensor retinaculum is attached to the radius, laterally and posteriorly, and to the ulna and hamate, medially. Its proximal border is under the distal crease of the wrist. The extensor tendons pass deep to it, i.e. extensor digitorum communis, extensor indicis, extensor digiti minimi, extensores pollicis brevis and longus, extensor carpi radialis longus and brevis, and extensor carpi ulnaris.

The *extensor tendons* can be seen on the posterior surface of the hand when the fingers are extended.

When the thumb is extended a depression is seen at its base, called the *'anatomical snuff-box'*. This is formed by the tendons of *abductor pollicis longus* and *extensor pollicis brevis* on the side of the thenar eminence, and the *extensor pollicis longus* posteriorly.

On the *palmar* surface of the hand, the *thenar eminence* (*see Fig.* 48) is formed by the muscles of the thumb (*abductor* and *flexor pollicis brevis*) laterally. The *hypothenar eminence* medially, at the base of the little finger is formed by abductor and flexor digiti minimi.

The *palmar fascia* covers the tendons of the fingers, in the palm, and has the palmaris longus tendon inserted into it.

VESSELS OF THE ARM

The *axillary artery* is a continuation of the subclavian artery, and enters the axilla at the level of the lateral border of the 1st rib. It becomes the *brachial artery* at the level of the lower border of the teres major.

With the arm abducted and the forearm supinated the

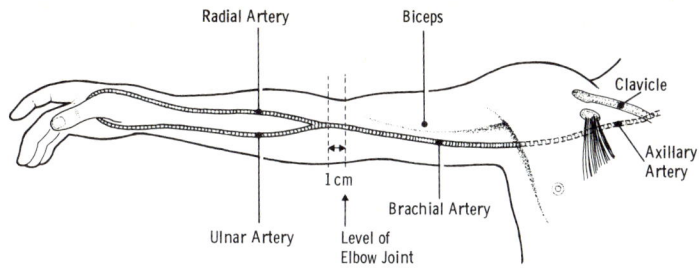

Fig. 50. Arteries of arm.

axillary, brachial and radial arteries lie on a straight line drawn from the centre of the clavicle to the styloid process of the radius at the wrist (*Fig.* 50).

The *axillary artery* can be divided into three parts:

1. From 1st rib (or centre of clavicle) to the medial border of pectoralis minor muscle; this is situated in the infra-clavicular fossa.

2. Beneath pectoralis minor; below the coracoid process.

3. Between pectoralis minor and teres major. It is covered by the pectoralis major and lies in the lateral wall of the axilla in the groove behind the coracobrachialis muscle.

The pectoralis minor muscle may be identifiable by its origin from the 3rd, 4th and 5th ribs and its insertion into the coracoid process.

The *brachial artery* extends from the lower border of teres major to a point 1 cm ($\frac{3}{8}$ in) below the elbow joint opposite the neck of the radius where it divides into *radial* and *ulnar arteries.* It lies at first medial to the humerus and then winds round medially, to lie in the midline between the humeral epicondyles, at the cubital fossa, just medial to the biceps tendon (*Fig.* 49).

The *radial artery* continues the main line of the brachial artery from the cubital fossa (*see above*) to become the deep palmar arch in the palm of the hand. 2·5 cm (1 in) above the level of the radial styloid process, the artery can be felt over

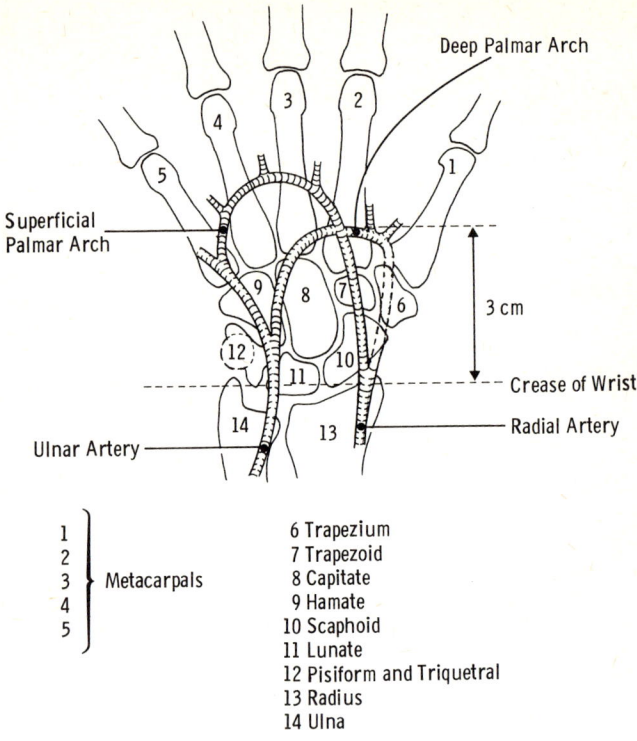

1 ⎫
2 ⎬ Metacarpals
3 ⎬
4 ⎬
5 ⎭

6 Trapezium
7 Trapezoid
8 Capitate
9 Hamate
10 Scaphoid
11 Lunate
12 Pisiform and Triquetral
13 Radius
14 Ulna

Fig. 51. Palmar arterial arches.

the lower end of the radius. The pulse is usually taken at this point. The artery winds around the lateral aspect of the wrist joint and carpus, lying on the floor of the 'anatomical snuff-box' overlying the scaphoid and trapezium posteriorly. It then passes through the space between 1st and 2nd meta-carpals to enter the palm of the hand. Turning medially it forms the *deep palmar arch*, anastomosing medially with the deep branch of the ulnar artery. The deep palmar arch is situated at a level 3 cm (1¼ in) distal to the distal crease of the wrist (*Fig.* 51).

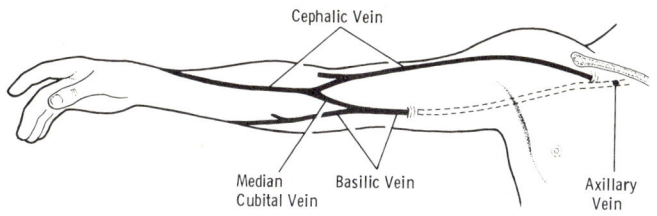

Fig. 52. Superficial veins of forearm.

The *ulnar artery* commences opposite the neck of the radius 1 cm (⅜ in) distal to a line joining the epicondyles of the humerus) at the bifurcation of the brachial artery. It lies on a line running medially from its commencement towards the medial epicondyle then turning downwards onto a line from the medial epicondyle to the pisiform in its distal two-thirds. It crosses into the palm of the hand superficially to the flexor retinaculum, and then divides into superficial and deep branches opposite the pisiform. The superficial branch forms the *superficial palmar arch* situated at the level of the cleft between the outstretched thumb, and the palm (*Fig.* 51). It supplies interosseous arteries to the fingers.

The deep veins of the arm all accompany the arteries, and have the same course and surface markings.

THE SUPERFICIAL VEINS OF THE ARM
Veins on the back (volar surface) of the hand drain into two main veins:

1. The *basilic vein* runs up the medial (ulnar) side of the forearm, commencing posteriorly then passing forwards to the anterior surface of the forearm below the elbow. The *median cubital vein* drains into it at the cubital fossa, and it then ascends along the medial border of the biceps brachii muscle, perforates the deep fascia, and drains into the axillary vein at the level of the lower border of teres major (*Fig.* 52).

2. The *cephalic vein* also commences on the dorsum of the hand, winding around the lateral (radial) border of the forearm

to ascend on the anterior surface to the level of the cubital fossa. Here it gives off the median cubital vein which crosses the cubital fossa obliquely in an upward direction, to join the basilic vein. The cephalic vein continues upward in the upper arm, between the deltoid and pectoral muscles, to reach the infraclavicular fossa. Here it pierces the coracoclavicular fascia to end in the axillary vein just below the clavicle (*Fig.* 52).

Chapter 13

The thigh and leg

1. MUSCLES OF THE BUTTOCKS AND THIGH

The buttocks are composed principally of the *gluteal muscles* (maximus, medius and minimus). These originate from the iliac crest and outer surface of the iliac bones and are inserted into the shaft and greater trochanter of the femur. They are responsible for keeping the body in an upright position by extending the hip joints; hence their large size and prominence (*Plate* 7).

Anteriorly, the folds of the groin correspond to the *inguinal ligament* (Poupart's ligament), below which, the front of the thigh is covered by the *quadriceps femoris* muscles, consisting of the *rectus femoris* (originating from the anterior inferior iliac spine and upper margin of the acetabulum), and the *vastus lateralis, intermedius* and *medialis,* which take origin from the shaft of the femur laterally, anteriorly and medially, respectively. They form together, the massive *quadriceps femoris tendon,* which is inserted into the upper border of the patella, and which can be felt in the lower thigh, above the patella (*Plate* 8).

The quadriceps tendon is continued below the patella as the *patella ligament* (ligamentum patellae) inserted into the tibial tuberosity at the upper end of the shaft of the tibia anteriorly. This, also, can be felt below the patella. The patella acts as a sesamoid bone in this tendon.

Crossing the quadriceps muscles, from the outer to the inner side (going downwards) is the *sartorius* muscle, originating from the anterior superior iliac spine, and inserted into the upper end of the tibia anteriorly. It can be seen under the skin, as a ridge crossing the thigh muscles. It forms the lateral

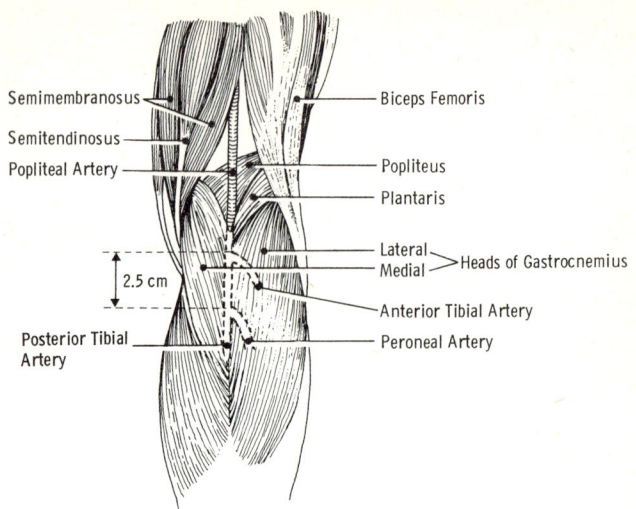

Semimembranosus

Semitendinosus

Popliteal Artery

Biceps Femoris

Popliteus

Plantaris

Lateral
Medial — Heads of Gastrocnemius

2.5 cm

Anterior Tibial Artery

Posterior Tibial
Artery

Peroneal Artery

Fig. 53. Popliteal fossa.

border of the *femoral triangle,* with the inguinal ligament above, and the *adductor muscles* on the inner side, completing the triangle.

Posteriorly, the *semimembranosus* and *semitendinosus* muscles, originating from the ischial tuberosity, on the medial side, and the *biceps femoris* laterally, all have tendons crossing the knee, inserted into the upper ends of the tibia and fibula posteriorly (the hamstring tendons).

The *popliteal fossa,* situated behind the knee joint, is bounded above by these tendons of semimembranosus and semitendinosus medially, with the tendon of biceps femoris laterally. Its floor consists of the posterior surface of the femur above, the posterior ligament of the knee joint (oblique popliteal ligament), and the *popliteus* muscle overlying the posterior surface of the tibia below. On either side, inferiorly, are the tendons of origin of the medial and lateral heads of the *gastrocnemius muscle (Fig.* 53).

On the medial side of the thigh, the *adductors magnus longus and brevis* originating from the pubic and ischial bones of the pelvis, are inserted into the medial posterior surfaces of the femoral shaft (*Plate* 8).

The *calf muscles* in the lower leg posteriorly, consist mainly of the gastrocnemius, originating from the femoral condyles by two tendons (as mentioned above) together with the *soleus* which takes origin from the posterior surfaces of the tibia and fibula. These muscles unite together to form the *tendo calcaneus* (tendo achillis), which is inserted into the posterior surface of the calcaneus (os calcis). This tendon can be seen and felt, behind the ankle joint (*Plate* 9).

Deep to these muscles are the flexors of the ankle and toes, also originating from the posterior surfaces of the tibia and fibula, and inserted into the tarsal bones, metatarsals and toes (tibialis posticus, flexors hallucis and digitorum longus).

These have tendons passing over the tip of the medial malleolus, which can be felt on the inner side of the ankle, and under the *flexor retinaculum.*

Between the tibia and fibula, are the *peroneus longus and brevis,* inserted into the tarsals and metatarsals, with tendons passing below the lateral malleolus (*see Fig.* 14).

Down the front of the lower leg are situated the extensors of the toes and ankle.

These consist of *tibialis anticus, extensors digitorum* and *hallucis longus,* which are inserted into the medial cuneiform and first metatarsal bones and the toes.

These tendons cross the front of the ankle, under the extensor retinaculum (anterior cruciate ligament).

The sole of the foot contains a strong fascia, the plantar fascia, and the *flexor muscles* of the toes (*flexors hallucis* and *digitorum brevis* and *accessorius*) *abductors hallucis* and *minimi digiti,* and *adductor hallucis obliquus.*

2. VESSELS OF THE LEG

The *femoral artery* is a continuation of the external iliac artery. It commences at the level of the midpoint of the inguinal

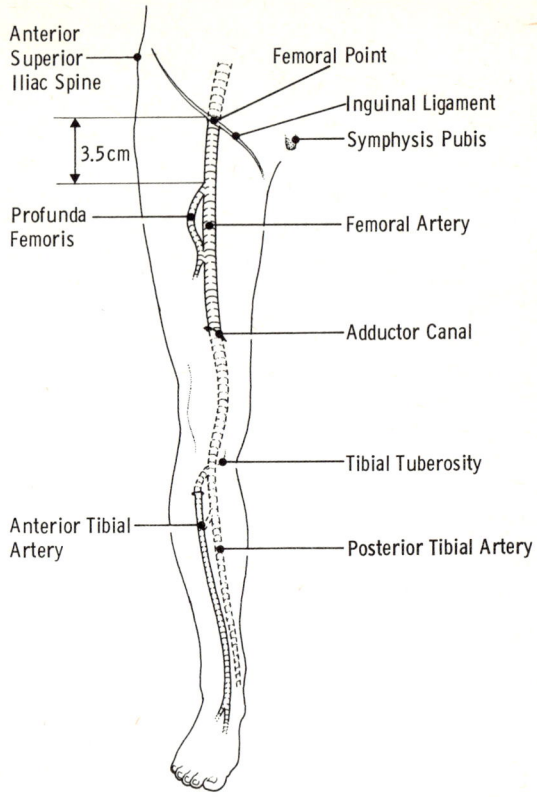

Fig. 54. Arteries of leg.

ligament (half way between the anterior superior iliac spine and the symphysis pubis) – known as the *femoral point* (*Fig.* 54).

The surface marking of the femoral artery is the upper two-thirds of a line from the femoral point to the adductor tubercle on the medial femoral condyle, curving around the inner side of the thigh. With the leg adducted, everted and knee flexed, this forms a straight line. Branches from the artery supply muscles in the thigh.

The *femoral vein* lies close to the medial side of the artery and then deep to it, lower down.

The *profunda femoris artery* arises 3·5 cm (1½ in) distal to the inguinal ligament, laterally. It winds around to the medial side of the femur, passing deep to the femoral artery, supplying muscles around the hip and on the medial side of the thigh. The *profunda femoris vein* accompanies it. Branches from the artery supply muscles in the thigh.

The *popliteal artery* is the continuation of the femoral artery, commencing at an opening in the adductor magnus muscle, which transmits the artery; situated at the junction of the middle and distal thirds of the thigh. The artery (together with the *popliteal vein*) crosses the popliteal fossa, to the lower border of the popliteus muscle, at the level of the tibial tuberosity, where it divides to form the anterior and posterior tibial arteries (*Figs.* 53 and 54). The surface marking of the popliteal artery in the popliteal fossa is on a vertical line from the upper end of the fossa, slightly medial to the midline, to a point opposite the tibial tuberosity.

The *anterior tibial artery* runs anteriorly to the front of the leg at a point half way between the head of the fibula and the tibial tuberosity. It can be represented by a line from this point to another point on the anterior surface of the ankle, midway between the medial and lateral malleoli.

It supplies branches to the knee and muscles of the front of the leg.

The *anterior tibial artery* becomes the *dorsalis pedis artery* at this point and then runs downward and forward on the dorsum of the foot to the proximal end of the space between the 1st and 2nd metatarsals. Here it penetrates this space to pass through into the sole of the foot, between the bases of the 1st and 2nd metatarsals, as the *deep plantar artery*.

The *posterior tibial artery* lies on a line down the midline of the lower leg posteriorly from the level of the tibial tuberosity to a point midway between the medial malleolus of the tibia

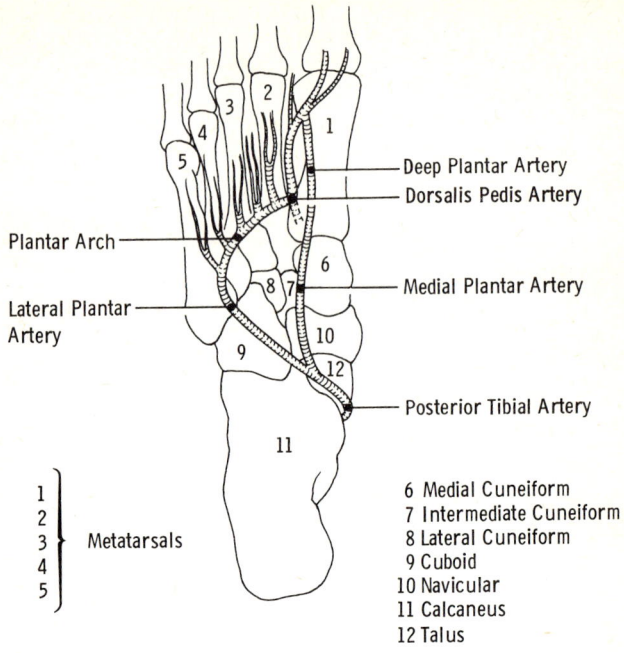

Deep Plantar Artery
Dorsalis Pedis Artery
Plantar Arch
Medial Plantar Artery
Lateral Plantar Artery
Posterior Tibial Artery

1
2
3 } Metatarsals
4
5

6 Medial Cuneiform
7 Intermediate Cuneiform
8 Lateral Cuneiform
9 Cuboid
10 Navicular
11 Calcaneus
12 Talus

Fig. 55. Plantar arterial arches.

and the tendo calcaneus. It can usually be felt at this point. The posterior tibial artery runs forward on the medial side of the foot, below the sustentaculum tali where it divides to form the *lateral* and *medial plantar arteries.*

The *peroneal artery* arises from the posterior tibial artery 2·5 cm (1 in) below the level of the lower border of the popliteus muscle and runs down the leg behind the fibula to the ankle.

The *lateral plantar artery* runs obliquely across the sole of the foot from below the sustentaculum tali to the base of the 5th metatarsal, where it turns medially, to become the *plantar arch,* supplying branches to the toes (*Fig.* 55).

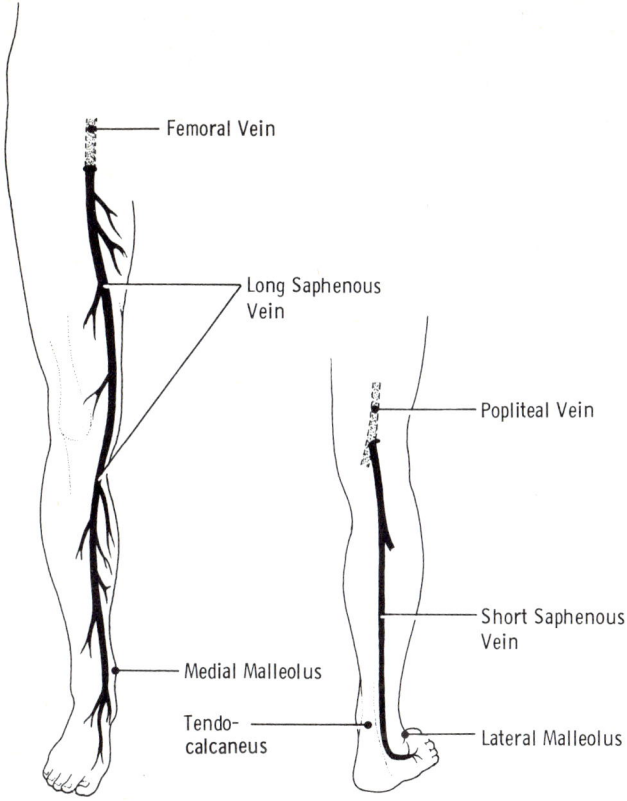

Fig. 56. Superficial veins of leg.

This plantar arch crosses the bases of the metatarsals from 5th to 1st, in the sole of the foot, and anastomoses with the deep plantar artery (the perforating branch of the dorsalis pedis — *see above*) (*Fig.* 55).

The medial plantar artery runs directly forwards along the medial border of the foot, to the great toe.

Corresponding deep veins accompany all these arteries.

3. SUPERFICIAL VEINS OF THE LEG

The short and long saphenous veins drain blood from the superficial venous networks of the foot.

a. The short saphenous vein arises on the lateral aspect of the dorsum of the foot, and passes up posteriorly in the calf of the leg, to the popliteal space, where it penetrates the popliteal fascia, to join the popliteal vein.

b. The long saphenous vein drains the medial border and medial aspect of the dorsum of the foot. It runs up the leg medially, behind the medial tibial condyle to join the femoral vein in the groin (via the fossa ovalis) under the inguinal ligament (*Fig.* 56). All these superficial veins have numerous valves preventing the reverse flow of blood down towards the feet.

Appendix Vertebral levels

Planes	*Landmarks*	*Structures*	*Vertebral Level*
		Base of skull	C1
			2
		Angle of mandible	3
		Upper border of thyroid cartilage	4
			5
		Cricoid cartilage	6
Thoracic inlet	Vertebra prominens	Lung apex	7
		Superior mediastinum	T1
	Suprasternal notch		2
			3
			4
	Sternal angle	Tracheal bifurcation	5
		Anterior and posterior mediastinum	6
			T7
			8
Xiphisternal plane	Xiphisternal joint	IVC opening in diaphragm	9
		Oesophageal opening in diaphragm	10
			11
		Aortic opening in diaphragm	12

Vertebral levels *(continued)*

Transpyloric plane	Middle of costal margin	Pylorus	L1
		Gallbladder	2
		Renal vessels	
		Head of pancreas	
Subcostal plane	Costal margin — lowest points	3rd stage of duodenum	3
Supracristal plane	Top of iliac crests	Aortic bifurcation	4
Transtubercular plane	Iliac tubercles	Ileocaecal valve	5
			S1
			2
			3
			4
			5
	Symphysis pubis	Tops of greater trochanters	
			Coccyx

Bibliography

Hamilton, W. J., Simon, G. and Hamilton, S. G. Ian. (1971) *Surface and Radiological Anatomy,* 5th ed. London, Macmillan.

Hartt, Fred, (1969) *Michaelangelo – The Complete Sculpture.* London, Thames & Hudson.

Kobayashi, Hellman, Fellisti and Cromb (1972) *Atlas of Ultrasound in Obstetrics and Gynaecology.* London, Butterworth.

Kramer, J. (1972) *Human Anatomy and Figure Drawing.* Wokingham, Van Nostrand Reinhold Co.

Lockhard, R. D. (1970) *Living Anatomy.* Faber & Faber Ltd.

Romanes G. J. (ed.) (1972) *Cunningham's Textbook of Anatomy,* 11th ed. London, Oxford Medical Publications.

Spalteholz, W. (1906) *Hand Atlas of Human Anatomy.* Philadelphia, Lippincott.

Warwick, R. and Williams, P. L. (ed.) (1973) *Gray's Anatomy.* 35th ed. London, Churchill Livingstone.

Wells, P. N. T. (ed.) (1972) *Ultrasonics in Clinical Diagnosis.* London, Churchill Livingstone.

Index